MW00965426

THE BRONZE KILLER
Marie Warder

The story of a family's fight against a very
common enemy

including
"IRON—the other side of the story!"
The layman's reference to Hemochromatosis
Canada's NO 1 GENETIC DISORDER

ISBN 0-88925-885-6

Printed in Canada

ABOUT THE WRITER.

BESIDES BEING THE FOUNDER AND NATIONAL PRESIDENT of the Canadian Hemochromatosis Society, Marie Warder is the author of 14 published books. At the age of seventeen she was, according to "The Journalist", the youngest chief reporter in the world. She sold her first newspaper article at the age of 11 and her first short story at 17.

All in all, it seemed that she had a good career ahead of her in her native South Africa, but, when a handsome, tanned young man in an air force uniform walked into the newspaper office one day, just before her 17th birthday, all ambition dissolved; she cared only about her "bronze soldier", as her mother referred to him. He was, from all accounts, endowed with "extraordinary physical strength" and was an excellent swimmer. When he returned from the war, the Mediterranean sun had deepened the tan to an even more magnificent bronze. The marriage took place when he was 21 and she 19. By that time Tom's father—who came from a handsome but short-lived family — had died, at the age of 50. . . . he just didn't come home from work one day!

The young couple worked very hard to establish themselves. Tom came to hold a responsible job with an airline; Marie wrote novels and qualified as a teacher, finally opening her own, private school of which she was the principal for ten years, prior to coming to Canada. Tom's dance band, in which Marie played the piano for 35 years, became exceedingly successful. They were riding the crest of the wave when disaster struck. The first indication was that Tom's eyesight deteriorated; his personality changed. The hypothesis she has given in the first chapter of "Iron— the other side of the story" could be an understatement of his experience.

As she tells in the book, "The Bronze Killer", they had come to the end of the good times. Little by little, their lives disintegrated. For six years, before doctors were able to diagnose his real problem, Tom grew sicker and sicker. His "sudden onset diabetes" advanced rapidly and he became progressively more resistant to insulin. Terrified as her " bronze soldier" became a "mahogany-coloured skeleton" before her eyes, she had to stand by, helpless, as he lost his eyelashes and body hair, his memory deteriorated and he became more and more confused. At last, the sickly slate grey colour, as she describes it, drew the attention of a knowledgeable doctor and—as she is fond of saying, "shades of Robin Hood!"— he was bled "a gallon of blood a month" to save his life.

At that stage, they could not be sure; too little was known and every member of the previous generation, who might have been a key, had died. There was, however, a possibility that their son would inherit the disease which had all but incapacitated his father; their daughter, everyone assured them, was safe. Tom's eyelashes had grown again, he had weathered severe spells of angina—which finally led to premature retirement—and even though he was no longer disoriented, he remained a "brittle diabetic" with increasing joint problems. They watched their boy like hawks.

Meanwhile, their daughter, her husband and children, had settled in Canada and, when Tom thought that he would die, he decided to bring his wife and son to this country—so that Marie would have the children around her when he was no longer there —but Visas took two- and- a- half years to obtain and Tom was still alive when they reached here.

They settled in Calgary where they soon made friends and were extremely happy — until another blow struck them. Their beloved daughter was diagnosed as having, as she told her parents, "this iron thing!" Blessedly the disorder had been detected in a very early stage, with no tissue damage, but she, too, would have to be bled regularly. Now, indeed, their lives could never be the same. They were overwhelmed by the implications as they realised what their daughter had been spared by timely diagnosis; they were terrified at what might await future generations—not only of their family but the families of others who were not similarly forewarned.

Today the whole family is involved in making Canada aware of the murderous potential of Hemochromatosis, the potentially fatal disease caused by an overload of iron. Their newsletter goes to hospitals, doctors and patients in nine countries. For four years, Marie and Tom have been travelling to various parts of Canada, talking on television and the radio; giving newspaper interviews. Her book will, she hopes, finally create the awareness for which they have worked so hard.

J.H.
March, 1988

In sincere gratitude to all those who help me "fight the bronze killer"—to the doctors who are doctors and the doctors who are patients; to the members of the Canadian Hemochromatosis Society—and in tremendous love and admiration for my "Exhibit A", who has lost so much. . . . and won so much!

INTRODUCTION

I HAVE BEEN BLESSED—AND HAVE BEEN SUBJECTED TO A great deal of anguish in the process—to learn much about the "Bronze Killer" in the years that have passed since I first began, in 1980, to try and record the bloody battle which my family has had to wage in trying to come to terms ("combat" and "vanquish" are not words to be employed in the confrontation) with this menace.

All that was known then, even by authorities on the subject, was—and still is—inadequate, and the only way anyone can hope to win in a fight against this thing is to strike early—before it does! Once you're literally gripped in mortal struggle, you're on your own—unless you're one of the fortunate few and meet up soon with someone who, recognizing the foe for what it is, can help you to make a stand when you're too weak to go it alone. Even then you'll engage in battle knowing, at the outset, that you will be required to shed gallons of your blood before the enemy evinces the slightest sign that you may be gaining ground.

From then on? Never relax your vigilance. . . . never turn your back on the relentless pursuer lest it creep up on you again and attack you unawares! Slay it? Not likely! The best you can hope for is to stun it; shock it into a state of suspended animation.

What's the answer then? There's only one: intercept it well before it rears its ugly head.

The knowledge that I have garnered, has made me realize that the very title is a misnomer, for the killer is not always evident, and then not really bronze. In my own imagination, the origin of this destroyer rears up as the true enemy, and it is that to which I now refer as the "Bronze Killer". As was the case with Dr. Frankenstein and his creation, one may well ask which is the greater monster? The cause or the effect?

I have ceased to be bitter, but there can be no dedicated Jew as ruthless in patient pursuit of the Nazi tormentor whom he has sworn to bring to justice, as I am in the crusade to expose the ravages perpetrated by IRON—this evil with its grinning mask of virtue. It is difficult to find an analogy which would convey the desperate urge which drives me. Such is my hatred of iron and my experience of its potential for destruction, given the right circumstances, that I will not give up until family physicians everywhere are on the lookout for, and know how to recognize Hemochromatosis; until the public are sufficiently alert to the danger of self-prescription to desist from this crazy practice of resorting to iron as a "cure-all" for everything from senility to impotence.

If I had my way, dietary iron would carry a warning label (after all, sensible people test the ph of a swimming pool before adding chemicals) and a Royal Commission would be appointed to study the effects of iron as a food additive. Blood tests for iron overload would become as common as a "Pap" smear—unless other tests had proven *conclusively* that a patient was iron deficient. Every victim of "sudden-onset" diabetes would be scrutinized for possible accumulation of iron, and, whenever a diagnosis of Hemochromatosis was made, all first-degree relatives of the victim would be screened. If everyone were as familiar with the word "Hemochromatosis" as with influenza, and potential sufferers were detected in time, much of the agony of a crippling and too often fatal disease would, within twenty-five years, become a thing of the past. As I never tire of stressing, we are talking about the most common of genetic disorders; yet Hemochromatosis remains, paradoxically the one about which 9 out of 10 people have never heard!

Until government and other health authorities recognize the prevalence of the disease, anything that can be done to combat it will remain ineffectual—and the desired, official recognition will not be forthcoming while medical advisers to the relevant authorities remain convinced that the problem is too rare to be of concern. In order to qualify for a tax number, so desperately needed for an organization which operates on a shoe-string, the Canadian Hemochromatosis Society was, for some years, precluded from engaging in activities designed to pressure government. Because of this, I have frequently become desperate enough to contemplate resigning from my position as National President in order to lobby in my personal capacity.

My inherent moral cowardice disperses when I am talking about iron and what it has done to my family and the families of so many people known to me. This is a blessing, as there have been some really disheartening times, and discouraging experiences by the score, since I first felt moved to tell this story. My voice has long not been loud enough for one crying in the wilderness. Only now are we beginning to see the results of ceaseless activity.

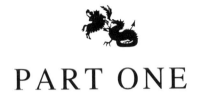

PART ONE

THE BRONZE KILLER:

CHAPTER ONE

IF I SAY THAT I HAVE HAD FOUR HUSBANDS WHILE REMAIN-
ing married to, faithful to and in love with the first—the true darling of my heart and the sweetheart of my youth—I do not mean
to give the impression that I have been indulging in polygamy.
The explanation is, in fact, relatively simple; my husband has
been all of these men. Through no fault of his own, Tom's personality underwent so many changes over a period of ten years,
that at times I had to cling almost desperately to the memory of
the man I had loved and who had shared my life for twenty-five
years before this. In order to tolerate the second personality, I had
to keep before me constantly the mental picture of the first.

Tom at nineteen, was extraordinarily handsome, possessed of
extraordinary physical strength and blessed with an extraordinarily beautiful body. He was a young man to make any girl's
heart beat faster but, apart from these outward and visible attrac-
tions, he was just thoroughly nice. Kind, gentle, patient and con-
siderate; the perfect young man, outrageously good-looking in
his Air Force uniform and I, at the age of seventeen, fell head-
over-heels in love at first sight.

None of what I have described—or ascribed to him—is ir-
relevant in the story; nor is it attributable to the sentimentality of
a loving heart who saw him through rose-coloured spectacles.

Everyone who knew him, loved him; he was the "catch" of
our town and hours of swimming or sailing his little yacht had

contributed to a magnificent tan which only enhanced the charm of flashing white teeth when he smiled.

I was nearly eighteen when he returned from the war: the tan deepened to mahogany. My mother teased my about my "Bronze Soldier", as she referred to him—in spite of the fact that his eyebrows and hair had been bleached to almost silvery gold—and she adored him. Although we were both so young she consented readily to our marriage which took place soon after Tom turned twenty-one.

He came from a long line of handsome, but notoriously short-lived men, and would make jokes about my having to appreciate him and make the most of every minute I had him, because he would "pop off at fifty!" Not long after we became engaged, Tom's father died—at the age of fifty. On Tom's fiftieth birthday he, himself, was in hospital with a life-expectancy of possibly twelve weeks.

But that is looking too far into the future. Soon after we were married, my new young bridegroom laughingly reminded me that he didn't have any time to waste, and our daughter was born just two months after his twenty-second birthday. He was a wonderful father and Leigh was the sort of child that could only result from a union such as this, in which there was so much love. She was an adorable, "golden" baby and has ever been a joy to anyone with whom she comes into contact.

We had to wait more than seven years for our second child, the much longed for and eagerly-awaited son, as I had several miscarriages in the meantime; but, although I was desperately disappointed and sad each time, we got on with the business of living and building up a home. Tom was with an airline and doing very well and, since we were both musical, and both played in the band of which Tom was the leader, there was enough money for us soon to have the type of home which was the envy of many people twice our age. The arrival of our son, Shaun, finally made our little family—and our happiness—complete.

A key to Tom's personality and success was the fact that he was so vibrant: so vital. He loved life with a capital "L". How he could burn the candle at both ends! Yet, he never neglected any duty, because he had such an abundance of energy and the resilience of excellent health. He could stand in front of the band for five hours on end—he would never sit down—and, by sheer force of his personality and infectious enjoyment, he would sweep us all along with him so that we played as we never believed we could and the crowd kept yelling for more. It was not long before the band was one of the most popular in our province.

By the time Leigh was twenty, Tom had risen high in his profession and we were travelling all over the world, making friends in many countries, and, wherever we went, it was always Tom's, healthy, tanned appearance that first made people notice him; and then his warm, friendly but gentle and sympathetic nature that endeared him to them.

I had a husband in a million and I knew it. I was almost smug about the fact and I enjoyed being the envy of friends. There were many who indeed envied me my husband, my lovely children and my style of life. We had a perfect marriage, a perfect family, a perfect gem of a servant, a perfect garden and a perfect home. In fact, our lives must have been as nearly perfect as any humans could wish for. We shared the same religious convictions and went faithfully to the beautiful church in which we'd been married, the children baptized and in which we hoped Leigh would someday be married and our grandchildren baptized. There we were surrounded by the love and friendship of others of our faith.

Meanwhile time had been creeping up on us. Our little Leigh, our golden, cuddly chicken had been growing up and changing into a lovely, serene young woman with a delicious sense of humour. She had never given us anything but pleasure, and when the time came for her to fall in love, she behaved as she would have been expected to do and delighted us by marrying the son of our best friends. Needless to say, both fathers-in-law were overjoyed and we mothers-in-law were as pleased as if we'd personally arranged the marriage to suit ourselves. Leigh, herself, had long been a friend and confidante-- often I forgot that she was my daughter—and her marriage strengthened our friendship and regard. For many years she and her husband had to be rocks upon whom all the family leaned.

In the August of the year in which his sister was married, and just before he, himself turned fourteen, we took Shaun to New York and he and I had the opportunity for sight-seeing while

Tom, who had to complete a course of instruction related to the new aircraft which the airline had purchased, attended lectures. The only bad memory of a happy holiday is that Tom kept complaining about his eyesight. During the long flight,there had been no pleasure for him in glancing at newspapers or magazines to pass the time, because he couldn't read them very well. Shaun teased him with veiled references to "advancing years" and "the march of time" but soon it wasn't funny any more because Tom was finding it difficult to see the blackboard and often didn't recognize his lecturers out of the classroom. It was decided that he would have his eyes tested as soon as we arrived home. When he could hardly see familiar people wave to him as they danced by at a wedding for which we played soon after our return, we knew he'd have to see about getting glasses.

It was not long after this that Tom began to exhibit all the classic signs of Diabetes: loss of weight, excessive thirst, exhaustion. Strangely, however, it took the doctors a long time to find out what was wrong with him and I wonder what would have happened if I hadn't read an article in the Reader's Digest and demanded that he be given a blood glucose test. This spelled the beginning of a major upheaval in our lives, but, fortunately, we didn't fully realize this at the time. Our doctor prescribed three tablets a day and Tom was told to watch his diet.

I read books and learned as much as I could about the disease—but no-one ever warned me about the terrible, unpredictable rages. Of all the people in the world, I was probably the most ill-prepared for temper which flared so quickly, or for fury that sometimes almost bordered on violence, for I had been the most cossetted and spoiled of wives. I had never known anything but love and gentleness and I was bewildered. To play in the band became sheer torture for all of us because we couldn't do a thing right. To go out visiting was no pleasure because, before long, Tom would do something wrong—or I would—and we'd argue all the way home.

To make matters worse, Tom, very markedly lost all interest in me. My presence seemed, in fact, to irritate him, and when we quarrelled there was never the joy of making up. He'd turn his back on me and I would cry, stormily and hopelessly until he'd be provoked to take notice of me. Then he'd snatch up his pillow with a furious: "For God's sake, do I have to lie here all night listening to that?" and go to bed in the adjoining room where he'd sleep so heavily that nothing, but *nothing* could rouse him.

That deep, awful sleep; that excruciating knowledge that, once he'd fallen into it, he was lost to me until morning! The fearful realization that I couldn't rely on him if a burglar came or the house burned down: How I hated that rasping snore and the severance it represented! How lonely the house was and how I missed my children!

Many a night, when the weather was warm, I would go and sit, sobbing beside the pool until the first light of day. Often I thought of hurling myself into the pool—the pool in which we no longer swam because we no longer had the heart for fun. Strangely, though, Tom still retained his deep tan and looked remarkably well. I was the one who looked tired and drawn.

In winter I used to crouch before the dying fire and sometimes I screamed out aloud in that cold, quiet house, hoping against hope for some response, even if it were only a reprimand.

Daylight would bring little relief because Tom would wake unrested and cross, and drag himself off to work to go and give everyone hell there—only I didn't know that at the time.

The next three years were the worst of my life. I was so unutterably lonely. And then I came at last to the dreadful conclusion that there must be another woman. Every time I asked Tom outright whether he still loved me, he would only snarl at me as though he loathed me.

My daughter was my strength and my fortress but I don't think she suspected more than that I was distraught about her father's poor health. As I was teaching at a private girl's school at the time and had every afternoon to myself, I went to her house most days, straight from school. She was joyfully awaiting her first child and glad, I like to think, of my company, but—for the very reason that she loved her father and me equally well and was secure in the thought that her parents had a perfect marriage—I could not confide in her. She was worried enough about Tom, as it was, and had the right to enjoy her pregnancy without the horrible suspicion that her father might be having an affair.

I spent a fortune in long distance calls to my sister, Claudia— but usually only discussed my concern about Tom's health. Pride would not allow me to tell anyone that my husband no longer wanted me. Whenever I carried to the doctor a list of numerous aches and pains which constantly beset me, or tried to tell him how irrational Tom had become, he would shake his head and give me tranquilizers which I would never take.

At school I had begun to turn inward so that I had to force myself to care about my pupils. I have never believed that teachers have the right to take out their own, private problems on their students, and I must have succeeded in putting on a very convincing act. One day, when I burst into tears in the principal's office, she was most taken aback. In her opinion, I was the last person in the world who might have reason to be unhappy. I wanted to sob it all out to someone, that I didn't want to go home to that awful house; that Tom had become an unpredictable stranger; that I was worried and needed help. But I could not. My principal had been our friend for many years and I could not so rudely shatter for her the beautiful illusion of our wonderful marriage. To talk to my mother or our priest seemed somehow disloyal to Tom. I had never before felt quite so desolate.

On the way home, I made a decision. Shaun was away at boarding school and, that very day, I would begin to set the machinery in motion to bring him home. What was the good of a son if you could not have his company when you were lonely? I would have to be ruthless, disrupt his studies in the middle of a school year, but I'd have someone to talk to. He could make new friends and settle down at a day school nearer home.

That was probably the worst, the most ill-advised thing I ever did. It was not difficult to arrange because Tom was all for peace at any price; and to Shaun's headmaster I put forward such a good case that he ended up trying to convince *me* that we needed the child at home! Shaun, moreover, was missing his father sufficiently to want to be closer to him.

If I'd had more sense, I would have realized that, under the circumstances, boarding school was the best possible place for Shaun at that vulnerable stage in his life. He had made a comfortable little niche for himself there—he was well-liked and had many friends—and he could have retained, inviolate, the image he cherished of a young, vital father who was always fun to be with, and of a mother who was the only suitable consort for such a prince among men.

How can I ever erase for him the memory of those years in which he was slowly, but surely, disillusioned; the times he had to listen to his parents bickering and be forced against his will to take sides? The motorcycle we bought him was hardly a compensation.

If I could ramble on interminably, I could go into detail about those terrible years—but why dwell now on all that horror when the memory of it has mercifully begun to fade? There are some agonizing hours, however, of which the remembrance obtrudes whether one recalls them voluntarily or not.

There was, for instance, the dreadful night when Tom, having worked late—and having, consequently, eaten later than usual—went into the bathroom where he sat down beside the basin to splash his face with water because he felt so ill; and, as the swiftly running tap swirled the plug into the outlet to seal it, he fell forward so that the rising water almost drowned him. With the aid of Jackson, our faithful servant and friend, Shaun and I dragged Tom, sopping wet and soon snoring stertorously, to his bed, and there we took turns to watch him all night in case this swoon was something more serious. We were so ignorant, really, in spite of all we'd read. The doctor, who cannot be blamed for never taking seriously the condition of a man who looked so remarkably well in spite of such severe loss of weight, had told us very little, and we didn't know whether oral treatment of Diabetes could give rise to the same sort of hypoglycemic coma as that sometimes induced by injections of insulin.

Then there was the ghastly night of Shaun's accident. I still shrink from having to remember how we looked for him all night, after he'd only gone to the corner store on the beloved motorcycle "to buy a comic", and the look on Tom's face when the police came at four in the morning to say they thought they'd found him. I can still recall, all too vividly, how waves of faintness and nausea kept washing over me in the hospital to which Shaun had been taken, unconscious, after a reckless motorist had come roaring through a stop sign. As we tiptoed between rows of people, some sleeping, some groaning, harvest of one night's gleaning on the highways, we peered in the gloom into one face after another, trying to establish which of them might be that of our son. I remember bending at last over Shaun in an agony of shocked recognition but I recall, most clearly of all, how, in his still delirious state, his lips so swollen that it was difficult to understand what he was saying, he kept asking: "Mom, will you still love me?" . . . Mom, I'm ugly now . . . Mom will you still love me?" —Foolish child! How could he doubt me? I loved him as never before! But my heart bled to think of the ravaged perfection of that handsome young face. . . .

CHAPTER TWO

THE MOST AWFUL MOMENT OF ALL, WAS WHEN I FINALLY saw myself for what I was. I think I began to grow up then, at the age of 43! For the first time I began to see around me—instead of only looking inward, and, when I did this, I realized at last how sick Tom was. I'd been too wrapped up in my own selfish sense of deprivation to perceive his fear or to interpret manifestations of his bewilderment; I had given no heed to what I had, subconsciously known all the time. In my desire to lean on my son, I had been blind to his, Shaun's, loneliness and mounting sense of insecurity and I'd been too self-centred even to question Leigh's reserves of moral courage, humour and unfailing wisdom on which I drew so relentlessly. I had parasitically sapped encouragement and courage from my sister when I had lacked the fibre to look my problems in the face.

The problems were still there, of course, but I took a vow that I'd lick them, no matter what. I would start with my own immaturity and I would not be satisfied until my children realized that, for the rest of my life, they had in me a mother and not another sibling—and I would grow in moral stature until Tom could sometimes lean instead of always being leaned upon. In the process, I'd hold up my memory of the old Tom as a shield while I helped him fight our mutual enemy, the sickness which had metaphorically shorn my Samson so that he roared lest he betray his weakness.

For I knew now that there was no human rival and I was sufficiently aware to be able to interpret Tom's fluctuations of mood.

As I became less demanding, his rages were less often directed at me, and when I wept, it was in secret. I wept for him and not *at* him. If he was unstable, it was because his Diabetes was not controlled, and I had to steel myself over and over against the nonchalance of our doctor as I tried to persuade him that this was the case. Joe was a very good doctor, and had he not known us for so long or had so vast a practice, he might have been more perceptive and open to conviction. He might have been more impressed by my insistence, as time went by, that this was no ordinary Diabetes which turned my Jekyll into a Hyde. During brief encounters, Tom usually managed to laugh and be pleasant to others and our doctor was deceived by this—as he was by Tom's still handsome tan.

In the circumstances, it has not been easy but, by the grace of God, by prayer and fasting—and, when necessary nagging or cajoling—I have tried when Tom has been too sick to do his own fighting, to keep the old devil, Disease, at bay for many years now. Some of his onslaughts have been devastating, however.

I gave our doctor no peace, as a result of which he increased Tom's tablets from three to four daily. Not long after this, the terrible diarrhea started. Nothing stayed in Tom's stomach for more than two hours. He lost more weight but continued to look remarkably well although painfully thin. Back I went to the doctor and tried hard not to notice that he, Joe, had by now to make a visible effort at patience, and I nagged again until stool cultures and other tests were done.

There seemed to be no remedy, no solution, no explanation for the debilitating diarrhea or the constantly high sugar.

Leigh's baby son was a great joy and consolation to us at that time and we took numerous photographs of him. Today those pictures are a lasting record, not only of our grandson's early progress, but of Tom's worsening health. Snapshots of him holding the baby, clearly show the toll the diarrhea was taking and, with his cheek against the baby's white skin, Tom's deep tan is quite startling by contrast.

Tom had to go to England on a course that year and Shaun and I went with him. How he managed at the factory, I do not know, because a walk down Oxford Street one Saturday afternoon was simply a desperate progression from one toilet to another. I am sure a lesser man would have succumbed by then. To make matters worse, although Shaun and I watched him like hawks and monitored everything he ate or drank, Tom's sugar remained alarmingly high in spite of the fact that there could never have been a drop of nourishment in his stomach. There was no doubt about it, the tablets were not controlling the Diabetes, and I began to suspect that they were the cause of the diarrhea.

On our return, I took advantage of the fact that Joe was on holiday, to tackle his partner—who did not know that I was supposed to be in the habit of "over-dramatizing"—and demanded that Tom be hospitalized immediately with a view to stabilizing him on injections of insulin. The results were absolutely astounding. I had taken to the hospital a mahogany-coloured scarecrow who had barely been able to tell us what day of the week it was, and I brought home with me a smiling, handsome, loving husband with whom I fell in love all over again. I felt as if my old Tom had come home to me after a prolonged absence; as I had known him before, but with a subtle difference. . . He seemed to be more self-effacing and, if possible, even more gentle and patient than he had been before. He went back to work, and it was only then that I began to hear from those with whom he worked, how pleased and happy *they* were at the metamorphosis. I could now fully appreciate what he must have had to suffer, knowing that he was alienating people of whom he was very fond—and how much they had been prepared to tolerate because of past regard for him.

His old exuberance soon returned and as the news spread that the band was once more available, we could have taken any number of bookings. We turned down many engagements, however, because we discovered that it was better being on the dance floor ourselves, instead of always performing on the stage.

What happy times those were. Tom was putting on weight steadily, now that his body could derive nourishment from what he ate, and the only problem was that he had to keep buying new clothes. For the first time we had our picture taken at a dance, among the dancers instead of with the band, and at this function—a "Gatsby" party—Tom can be seen looking better than he had done in years. The magnificent tan is very much in evidence.

Shaun, his wounds—literal as well as figurative—wonderfully healed and his scars almost imperceptible, had been called up for duty in the Air Force and looked almost as good in his uniform as his dad had before him. When Leigh's little daughter was born—another "golden" baby to delight us—we seemed to have weathered the storm and were completely happy once more.

The enemy was not prepared to relinquish its grip without another struggle, however. It soon transpired that when we did play, Tom could not stand in front of the band as he used to do in the old days, without suffering such severe cramps in his legs that we often had to stop the car on the way home. One night they came on so badly after we had already fallen asleep, that he very nearly blacked out from the pain and could not walk the next day.

Very soon after that I began to perceive other symptoms which were disquieting and, always a moral coward, I was a bit shy about being too persistent with either of the two doctors whom I'd previously consulted and who were clearly not over impressed when I presented them with a list of signs and symptoms which seemed to them to exist solely in my imagination. Consequently I waited for a suitable time when I could make an appointment with another doctor—Eric, the third member of the practice, who had only recently returned to our town—and that was the best thing I ever did. Somehow he took me seriously right from the start and listened with interest to all that I told him. From that day onward, he became our very good friend as well as our adviser; he and his wife were pillars of strength in time of trouble. If either of them should ever read this, where they have now settled in far away Saskatchewan, I hope that they will accept this tribute as an expression of our gratitude.

At last I had found a doctor whom I could approach directly without having to prepare my case like a lawyer fighting for the life of his client and facing a difficult jury. He always gave the impression that he considered my observations sensible and my concern reasonable. If Tom's condition was worsening at an alarming rate, it certainly was not for lack of care on the part of our doctor. He was not easy in his mind, from the start, about a "late onset diabetes" which, instead of being simple to control and possibly improving after the initial loss of weight, was clearly bolting along like a wild horse out of control.

For the wonderful improvement in Tom's health after he was first stabilized on insulin, was short-lived. It was not long before the dosage was increased and increased again, until he was on a maximum dosage twice a day. He was allergic to certain kinds and suffered all manner of rashes and lumps and bumps until we tried pork insulin. Some sort of atrophying process had by now caused a dent, the size of a man's fist, in his stomach muscles and half of one buttock seemed to have disappeared. His memory was failing and he was given tablets to try and stimulate his brain, which terrified him. Once over six feet tall, he had shrunk three-quarters of an inch.

Leigh and Bruce, my son-in-law, were preparing to emigrate to Canada and settle in Toronto with their little family, when I first learned that Tom had wide-spread arterio and atherosclerosis of the aorta; and, because she was so worried, Leigh and I— separately and together—consulted as many doctors as we could, without Tom's knowledge. One of them, upon looking at the X-rays we produced, pronounced them to be those of "A man of seventy"! --Tom was then nearly forty-nine. Another said he could hold out no hope while yet another comforted me with the assurance that he could do a by-pass. All were in agreement on one score: "This man's case is hopeless any way unless he gets that Diabetes under control... !"

By the time Leigh and Bruce left, it seemed as if Tom's sugar had been more or less stabilized on a mixture of insulins and Shaun was home from the Air Force, so that Leigh could go away reasonably reassured. The respite was a short one, however, and from then there was only one way and that was downhill. Tom could no longer make jokes about "popping off at fifty." We had then reached the stage when, although we did not realize it, his life-expectancy was about twelve weeks.

A month before his fiftieth birthday, Tom had become almost totally resistant to insulin. How he still went to work, I do not know. He could only walk with difficulty and was often very confused. One Sunday afternoon we went for a drive to the airport where there was an impressive line-up of international aircraft. There he could see, silhouetted against the setting sun, the tails of the planes he loved so well. It was a poignant moment and suddenly I saw a tear slide down his cheek. I knew that he was very weak and discouraged, but this was the first time in all our married life that he had ever openly betrayed such emotion or fear to me.

I had to try very hard to be strong, myself, when he said, "We have to face it Ma... This is the end of the line. There is no cure for this and I've got to accept it!"

He had often called me "Ma" since Shaun was born. Now, however, it was as if I were indeed the mother and he the child. And suddenly, at that moment, I felt a strength and confidence such as I had never known before, surge through every fibre of my being. We were *not* giving in yet!

"No," I agreed, and I knew that I spoke the truth. "There is no cure—*but there's God!*"

We had often talked about the miracle that *could* happen. Now I knew that it *would*—and it did... Not just one. To use a collective noun beloved of my grandchildren, a whole bunch of them!

Two weeks later, in Johannesburg, South Africa, Tom was sick enough to be admitted to the Diabetic clinic at the General Hospital there. The once splendid tan had become a sickly blue-grey pallor by then and, by some wonderful chance, the doctor to whom Tom was assigned, a lecturer at the university and a man intensely interested in skin pigmentations, was immediately arrested by Tom's remarkable colour. He was willing, he said, to stake his reputation on the diagnosis that the underlying cause of all that ailed my husband was an excess of iron in the system.

There were many factors—not least among them the rapid advance of maturity-onset Diabetes, the decreasing response to insulin and the bronze colour which we'd always associated with Tom—which pointed to a condition called Hemochromatosis; more commonly known in North America as "Bronze Diabetes". Some people accumulate an overload through ingesting too much iron—as is the case with many African tribes who cook in rusty iron pots—but there was much to indicate that Tom's Hemochromatosis was hereditary. As there was not even one of his uncles alive to testify, it could only be surmised that one or all of those handsome, "tanned" men who had died so young, were victims of the same killer—even if the method of attack had varied. Possibly Tom's father, whose death had been ascribed to "heart failure" at fifty, had died as a result of the same condition; for one does not die specifically of Hemochromatosis but because the iron lodges in a vital organ where it does untold damage.

It so happened that, right there at that hospital, at the right time and at the right place, there was a professor who was regarded as a world authority on this condition and he was very soon able to confirm the diagnosis. Liver and bone marrow biopsies were done, a deferinisation test was conducted and at last I knew why Tom had Diabetes. By then much of the damage was irreversible, for Tom's pancreas had virtually been destroyed by the iron which had collected there and his liver was badly damaged; but treatment would commence immediately and, after two years, there would be a significant improvement. It was because of the damage to the liver and possibly many glands of the endocrine system that he had no eyelashes, no hair on his legs and no chest hair.

Meanwhile, I thought, it was all very well talking about two years into the future if they couldn't keep him alive to begin the treatment, for he was almost comatose from the high sugar and completely resistant to every form of insulin which was tried—until the next miracle occurred... A firm in Scandinavia sent a small batch of experimental, monocomponent insulin to the hospital to be tested, as a last resort, on a woman who was dying. They decided to share this between her and Tom. Both of them responded and for at least a year—until this insulin came on to the market in its smart bottle and packaging—we were given it free of charge, simply by showing the letter they gave us, in any country where this laboratory had a depot. Once in Holland, at the beautiful Marriott Hotel in Amsterdam, the precious vial went missing from the hotel refrigerator and a taxi was dispatched after-hours to fetch the employee who'd last handled it. . . . But that's another story.

When anyone has Hemochromatosis, there is no way of ridding the system of the excessive iron except by a long-term program of bleeding. No transfusion is given because that would simply be exchanging new blood for old, and this would not eliminate the iron deposited in vital organs. In lay terms, the idea is to create iron-deficient anemia to the extent that the body is forced to feed on this excess iron in order to replenish its supply of blood; thus inducing its own cleaning up process.

Before the first "bleed", Tom was photographed in colour, cheek to cheek with a young woman doctor who had a very pale skin, so that those dedicated people would have a pictorial record of his diminishing "tan", and then he embarked on what was to become a way of life. In the beginning he had to be bled twice a week, a pint a time—which is the same as saying he was bled a gallon a month. I was sure no-one could survive this but, as the professor told us, "Hemochromatotics" make up that blood at an alarming rate, and for some time Tom experienced the "feeling of increased well-being" which the professor promised us. As soon as tests showed that Tom's iron level had decreased,he was told that one pint a week would be sufficient and, as we'd also been promised, there was a marked improvement after that initial two-year period.

It is this bleeding or "phlebotomy" and insulin—by the Grace of God, of course—which have kept him alive now for many years beyond that awful, half-century "popping-off" time; twelve years longer than his father was blest to enjoy. In spite of weakness which began to succeed the bleeds as the iron saturation diminished, during the two years following the diagnosis of his basic problem, Tom continued to hold down his job and did some of his best work, which included many inventions and improvements to aircraft flying throughout the world.

The most difficult part of the whole situation, proved to be the fact that few doctors anywhere else in the world had ever seen a case of Hemochromatosis. We had endless trouble trying to organize the bleeds in other cities. In Toronto, the doctor whom we finally persuaded to "do" Tom at one of the hospitals, admitted frankly that, until that moment, Bronze Diabetes had only been an examination question to him. He doubted that Tom really had it until we showed him the letter we carried. In Johannesburg they'd had a Hematology clinic where, as more cases were discovered, patients came to be bled on a routine basis but in Calgary, for instance, there was no such clinic and, on our first visit to that city, we had to keep' phoning around until we were referred to a specialist who agreed to do the phlebotomy. In desperation I had even tried to inveigle a lady at a Red Cross blood donor clinic at Chinook Mall to help us but, of course, as they did not want the blood, she was not prepared to bleed a man just to throw that pint away.

Then came the time when Tom began to have the most agonizing attacks of angina. . . perhaps from the constant dehydration; who knows? He could hardly walk from his car to work and repeated bouts of nocturnal angina robbed him of rest. He was given nitro-glycerin tablets to place under his tongue, but after two successive nights when the longest respite between attacks was twenty minutes—during which he'd doze, sitting on the edge of the bed and leaning forward to rest his head on the pillows we'd piled up on the dresser—he ended up in the intensive care ward. It was there that my nephew comforted me by saying, "He's not done yet, Aunty. He must be one of the strongest men I've ever known." And it was there that I began to wonder about this very thing.

Referring to his Diabetes, of course, Tom had always called himself my "sugar daddy", and soon after he learned that he had Hemochromatosis, he tried to make light of it by saying, "Well, Ma, you've got more than a sugar daddy now—you've got a man of iron!" This made me wonder about others who have this condition and whether it was, indeed, the excessive iron in his system which had given Tom his extraordinary strength and the zest for living which had characterized him as a young man. Did other incipient Hemochromatotics share these attributes before they were felled, in their prime, by this Bronze Killer?

I was so grateful to God for leading us to those who had discovered this thing which had threatened Tom's life, that I wished passionately to do something for others who might be similarly menaced and who could be spared untold suffering—or even death—by being forewarned and thus forearmed; by possibly becoming blood donors at an early age, before the iron saturation reached dangerous levels, serious damage could be prevented. I wrote numerous letters to cousins, warning them to have themselves and their children tested. I made countless telephone calls, wrote to doctors and "people in high places" urging that transferrin saturation and ferritin tests become a routine procedure after a certain age, and certainly in cases where people have developed sudden-onset Diabetes—but no-one would take me seriously. Relatives could not be frightened by what seemed sheer hypothesis—for who could really prove that Tom had inherited this condition? Others had never heard of this sickness or their physicians dismissed it as "being far too rare to bother about!"

Doctors who had never seen a case of Hemochromatosis protested that to requisition for the iron profile routinely would be superfluous, as the diabetic patient's colour would be sufficient indication of the presence of excessive iron.—Why then wasn't anyone disturbed by Tom's classic mahogany tan until he was almost at death's door?—Meanwhile it is almost impossible to buy a breakfast food or a night-time beverage which is not routinely "fortified with iron". I have read dozens and dozens of books on nutrition and only during the last few years has any writer made any mention of Hemochromatosis and the dangers of self-prescription of iron. Wherever I go, I make contact with the local branch of the Diabetic Association and am generally dismissed as a bit of a crank. One doctor, on learning that Tom has Hemochromatosis, could only ask: "Why? Is he an alcoholic?"

I began to be obsessed with the knowledge that some sort of foundation would have to be established to study this condition in Canada and I wanted more people to be aware of it. Often as my enthusiasm for the crusade began to wane, something would happen to make me want to try again—as was the case when Tom's feet became too painful for him to come for a walk with me,or it became increasingly difficult for him to play music because of the ache in his hands.

To counteract the effect of such drastic bleeding and to prevent the ensuing attacks of angina, it was decided that he should be given a saline drip. At one hospital, however, someone gave him a glucose drip by mistake and nearly killed him. Then I was mad enough to write some more letters—as I was motivated to begin writing *this*... !

Tom had fought valiantly for many years, but the angina was what finally brought about his "premature" retirement. In 1978 he, Shaun and I settled in Calgary where we were fortunate to find a family doctor who knew something about Hemochromatosis and was interested to know more. He put us in touch with an endocrinologist at the Foothills Hospital, who would do regular tests to ensure that Tom's condition was not retrogressing, and arranged with yet another specialist to undertake weekly phlebotomies at the Rockyview Hospital. He also dealt sympathetically with my concern about Shaun—for I had developed the habit of stealing into my son's room at night, when he was asleep, to see whether his face was looking too brown against the white pillow.

We remained painfully ignorant and there was no source from which we could obtain reliable information. We had been told in Johannesburg that it could be expected that two out of three sons might inherit this condition. Tom had had a brother who had died at birth; so we hoped that he might have been the other in that generation, for nothing we could do or say could persuade Selby, his other brother, to take this thing seriously. We also knew that the condition did not necessarily manifest itself as Bronze Diabetes: the liver is always in danger.

Not all the snippets we had gleaned, were necessarily correct. Someone had said erroneously that one male child would have a tendency towards alcoholism and I thought, almost gratefully then of the babies I'd lost, and prayed that they might have been the ones and not Shaun. About Leigh we were not in the least worried because we had been assured that she was not at risk. Hemochromatosis, had been detected in few women, as they menstruate and are consequently rather inclined towards anemia. Those who had been known to suffer from Hemochromatosis, it was said, had undergone hysterectomies or had developed the condition after the menopause.

Our son-in-law's work had taken him to Vancouver Island, and it was a welcome respite from the snows of Alberta to visit the little family whenever we could get away for a long weekend. At Thanksgiving we thought our little golden girl was looking a bit tired but revelled so much in the company of their two enchanting golden children—hardly babies any more—that we had little opportunity for a closer look.

Then, just before Christmas, 1979, Leigh 'phoned and said to her father, in a small voice but typically matter of fact manner: "Dad, it seems I've got this iron thing! And what could I say when he told me but, "Oh, my God!"

I felt as if I'd been dealt a mortal blow. I could neither sleep nor eat. Spectres and phantoms walked with me whichever way I turned. My imagination almost killed me... My darling girl, with her delicious sense of humour, thirty-one years old and possibly suffering a change of personality. My beloved son-in-law living through what I'd had to face!... Leigh having the ghastly liver and bone marrow biopsies; having, like Tom, to be bled for the rest of her life! I was so sorry for myself that I almost forgot to be sorry for her!

My sister pleaded with me not to take it for granted that Leigh's case was going to be a parallel of Tom's. Again I resorted to prayer and began to get things in the right perspective. Sure, Leigh did have to have the biopsies about which I'd agonized, and they proved that her iron saturation was abnormal—95% whereas a normal woman's might be around *25%*-there *was* a horrific amount of iron in her liver *but there was no tissue damage as yet.* How thankful we should be that she, by the Grace of God, lived in a place where there was a doctor who knew enough and cared enough for the condition to be detected *before* the real damage was done. He, in turn, had handed her over to the care of a specialist who knew a great deal about Hemochromatosis and what to do for her: She did not *have* to develop Diabetes and now that we had proof knew, beyond a shadow of a doubt that the "iron thing" was hereditary, steps could be taken to protect her children. She had a specialist who knew what he was doing.

There was no keeping me in Calgary after this and we lost no time in selling our home and moving to Victoria. The first time my two went off to be bled together, Leigh said to Tom: "The doctor must be glad you've come, Dad. It would have been a shame to break up the set!

CHAPTER THREE

One day in 1980, I made this entry in my diary:
Vancouver Airport South
October 23

WHAT A HELL OF A PLACE TO BE WRITING ONES "MEM-
oirs"! What a hell of a place to be, anyway! In a motor home,
parked in among a collection of helicopters and small aircraft, far
from home with nothing to do but this!

I've been in some strange places in my life and done some
weird and wonderful things—but this must surely take the cake!
Lucky we have this little R.V.. We call it the *"Hamba Gahle"*,
which is Zulu, I guess, for "Go Carefully". Everyone refers to it
simply as "The *Hammy*".

Because I hurt my back in April, lifting a vacuum cleaner at
work, I have been unable to sit comfortably in a car, and Tom
bought the *Hammy* so that we could at least get from point A to
point B with relative ease. We never thought it would become our
home—or that we'd live in it HERE! When Claudia came to visit
us last month, we took her to Calgary in it and she was absolutely
intrigued. She just couldn't get over it that I could travel from
Vancouver Island to Alberta, flat on my back!

The day after we saw her off, while she was still on her way
back home, Tom was starting work with a company here at the
south end of Vancouver Airport. We have permission to park

here during the week. On Fridays we go back on the ferry to Victoria.

Aircraft noise doesn't bother me; I've been accustomed to it all my married life and only wake up when something is different. (Tom likes to tell people that I jump out of bed at three in the morning, shouting: "Air Canada's late!")

No, it's not the place that's getting me down. I'm probably just feeling a bit bereft after weeks of such close contact. We had an unforgettably happy time together in the *Hammy*, the three of us; and now my beloved sister is halfway around the world from me and Tom has gone back to part-time work after all these years.

I worry about him. I guess that's natural after the way I've had to take care of him for so long. The only way I can describe how I feel, is to remember what it was like when the children started school; except only I'm a lot more anxious. It's fortunate that he has only ten yards to walk to the department in which he works and can come back at frequent intervals for a snack. When he does, I inspect him with a metaphorical magnifying glass. . . . on the alert for any sign that this new undertaking might be too much for him.

Then, when he goes back inside, the *Hammy* closes in around me. I'm used to living at five thousand feet above sea level. The sun shines brightly in Johannesburg, even in midwinter, and the interminable rain here can be positively claustrophobic.

When the windows mist over, I'm completely shut in. I'd love to be in my little house in Victoria, polishing the beautiful furniture I brought thousands of miles to make a home in this new country; but I still have Tom, which is a miracle, so I pass the time as best I can.

Sometimes, I jog along the river bank, or I wander through the terminal at Airport South. I spend a great deal of time at the pay phone, yearning to hear Leigh's voice. When I have spoken to her, I'm refreshed; renewed in mind and spirit. She has this effect on me; the ability to make problems diminish and heartaches vanish. . . . except when she is part of the heartache. . . !

Ever since she told me about herself, there has been this pain inside of me. It isn't really Air Canada that makes me leap out of bed, shouting, but I hope I convince Tom that it is so. He hurts about her, too, and it would make it worse if he knew how intensely I suffer.

No sooner was I able to make myself believe that it was true, than I began to agonize about other young people like her. I felt that I had suddenly become every mother; that my knowledge had placed upon me the responsibility for those who don't know. I still feel that way, but there's so little I can do.

In the first flush of crusading. I have written letters—none of which was printed—to numerous newspapers, and an impassioned article which I have submitted to most of the influential magazines in Canada. Reputable publications, it seems, seek expert advice before printing stories of this kind and, since those "experts" have not done their homework, the consensus of opinion is (a) that I am a crackpot or (b) that the disease I write about is "too rare to be of interest to the general public". The editor of a glossy weekly infuriated me by suggesting that we were to blame for not going to the right doctors in the first place. Which "medical help of the right sort" were we supposed to have sought?

Chatelaine at least showed me the courtesy of giving the manuscript a second reading, asking that it be re-submitted, after an initial rejection. The second response was the same as the first, however, and they're probably right. I'm not going to get anywhere until I have some case histories to substantiate what I say!

Meanwhile, here I sit, trapped in the *Hammy*. I've decided to write this book, to pass the time, but it's proving to be more difficult than I anticipated. After fourteen fairly successful novels, this should be easy. I thought I'd had sufficient training and had acquired the right degree of self-discipline for the task. I was wrong. Each night, as I read through what I have written that day, I recognize an element of sentimentality; emotionalism comes creeping through in spite of myself.

I try hard to rephrase and eradicate the weakness, but then I ask myself: how does one relate how the person one loves best in the world was rescued from death on the very brink of the grave—without becoming emotional?"

Because she is so tiny, it was not possible to bleed Leigh twice a week as had initially been done for Tom, but even one phlebotomy a week was hard for such a small body to take. She proved a difficult person to get blood out of as, I would someday learn from others, is sometimes the case in the early stages of treatment. Often, after three or four punctures, the doctors resorted to hot compresses. Eventually an anaesthetist was asked to perform the venesection (another term for the procedure) and he undertakes her phlebotomies to this day.

I was constantly distressed about her. To see her with her blouse or sweater spattered with blood was an agony. She would have to take to her bed after the blood-letting on a Tuesday, would feel weak until about Friday, and would then recover sufficiently to do her housework on a Monday—only to start all over again on Tuesday. She, however, insisted that she could only be grateful when she thought of the terrible suffering many people with other diseases have to endure. I worried about the children and her husband, but soon had proof of what I had suspected all along—that I have the best son-in-law in the world.

There finally came a day when my prayers were again answered and Leigh's blood tests showed such a dramatic—and miraculous—improvement that she was told she would only have to be bled once a month.

Once again I was inspired to take up the crusade; I was motivated once more to tackle the book. Perhaps it would move people to start asking questions or even stimulate further research. I would make another attempt.

I now had my daughter able to help me. Not only was she perhaps the youngest person in the world known to have this condition; she was living proof that Hemochromatosis is hereditary and that female offspring *can* inherit it—except in cases where it has been induced. I laid great emphasis on her colouring to make it known that there does not have to be that extraordinary tan to betray the build-up of iron in the tissues. Because she was born when her father was so young, they were both alive, simultaneously, to prove and disprove many hypotheses.

We would learn a great deal about HH in the years that lay ahead; we would get to know many other victims—younger and older—than Tom and Leigh were then; people with complications and manifestations vastly different from those which had touched our family. At that time, however, Leigh felt as I did. If her early diagnosis was indeed unique, she was extraordinarily fortunate; it was almost a sacred trust to make others aware of what she had tried to play down to her father by alluding to it as "this iron thing and its ramifications". Tom considered himself privileged to have been the guinea pig and thus instrumental in prolonging her life. If she had been frightened—and having to be a witness to her father's suffering, she must have been terrified—Leigh had never shown it, but she frequently expressed her gratitude for the fact that her father's experience, and hers, would protect her children.

We continued to fear for Shaun. And how ardently I wished that someone had known about the recessive gene which ran like a thread through this family, when Tom was young and could have been treated. Even before that, when his father and uncles might have benefited from the knowledge. Now I wondered whether Tom's Aunt Maisie (who, although suspected of being diabetic, had never featured previously in our conjecture because "it is unlikely that a woman will have it") had, in fact died of "kidney failure". What of Ella, my favorite among the Warder aunts—she of the bronzed skin—who had ended her days in a wheel chair, crippled with joint disease?

Tom held on to the job at Vancouver Airport for as long as he could, but the odds against that arrangement were really almost insurmountable. Not only were we both soon worn out by the constant rush of going to and fro; the ferry fare ate up nearly all his earnings. There was very little work on Vancouver Island for someone with Tom's qualifications. If we wanted to be able to live in our home in Victoria, *I* would have to find a job.

Before emigrating to Canada, I had held a wide variety of jobs. I had trained primarily as a journalist; then as a teacher. At one stage, after a miscarriage which had left me thoroughly demoralized, I had taken the advice of my doctor who recommended a "change of scene"—and had gone to work as the assistant to the services manager of the local head office of an international pharmaceutical company.

In the beginning, I was given only press releases to translate; then package inserts, labels and, occasionally the detailing literature—which was what the reps handed out with products. I checked proofs of all advertising and the time came when I was allowed to write some of the copy myself. My speciality was *monilia*, and I bet I could still turn out a pretty mean essay on *candida albicans!*

There was one task I enjoyed above all others, however. As medical publications came via my desk, it was my responsibility to go through them with a fine tooth comb, and to mark for the attention of the relevant manger or director such items as were pertinent to our products or field of research. At first I scanned the pages with an eye only for what I had been instructed to find; but by degrees, particularly as the subject matter became more comprehensible, I found myself reading with heightened interest. I became more and more fascinated, intrigued, caught up in what those pages revealed, until I was almost consumed.

Before long, I fell into the habit of taking films home, and watched them over and over until I knew enough about the subject matter to be able to reply with comparative authority to inquiries from medical practitioners and, in time to make the occasional recommendation. I loved my work and eagerly absorbed all I could learn from it; never dreaming how valuable that experience would someday be; never realizing how useful a knowledge of medical terminology would prove.

Because I was so happy in my job, I still don't know what moved me to leave. Almost as though I were a pawn on a chessboard or a piece on Omar Khayyam's "checkerboard of nights and days", after having been invited to go elsewhere, I found myself, in due course, the public relations officer of the Southern African operation of one of the worlds largest food companies; writing news releases; negotiating with people at executive level; speaking in public on a regular basis; interviewed by the media. The clay of my life was further being shaped by the master potter. It was a strange state of affairs: I was the public relations officer of a company which, in turn, retained a public relations company to promote *me*. The firm capitalized on the publicity I received as my books continued to sell and the growing popularity of Tom's band. I became South Africa's "Betty Crocker".

Then suddenly, I was felled like a tree; crippled to the extent that I had to undergo a miracle of surgery—an anterior spinal fusion—which necessitated major abdominal surgery to enable the orthopaedic specialist to reach my impaired backbone from the front. This meant three months in a plaster cast—with only my arms, head and legs (from the knees down) sticking out like those of a turtle from a shell. I lay flat on my back and learned to drink through a plastic tube. Because nothing would go down unless I chewed it, I chew even ice cream to this day.

With the aid of mirrors and numerous gadgets which Tom made for me, I carried on with my work as best I could; keeping up a correspondence with thousands of customers, users of the company's products, who had been exhorted to write to me, by the label on every can of coffee and the recipe cards in every canister or package of tea.

I guess that was good training for the mountains of letters I have to deal with now!

Since my arrival in Canada, I have come up repeatedly against the obstacle of "over qualification". I was eventually obliged to fall back on what had been my hobby and has become my bread and butter. . . . music.

And it was music that got us back home to Victoria. I was offered a job managing a piano and organ store, and Tom did the servicing—between phlebotomies and cardiograms; walking a tightrope between high sugar and hypoglycaemia. He became an increasingly brittle diabetic.

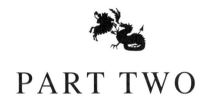

PART TWO

RETALIATION

CHAPTER ONE

Richmond, British Columbia

THE CANADIAN HEMOCHROMATOSIS SOCIETY BECAME A reality in 1982 and, one year later, our first newsletter was produced in Victoria, with Leigh's assistance. We already had one charming young volunteer called Debbie Norton, to help with typing. After all those years of seemingly getting nowhere, I could hardly believe that the society had finally been incorporated. It had taken months and months of skimping and scraping to raise enough money to start, about $300 worth of phone calls to Ottawa, two trips to Vancouver and repeated, discouraging visits to the local 'societies branch', until we finally had all the flaws in the constitution ironed out to everyone's mutual satisfaction.

Just after we were accepted for incorporation in November, 1982, I was interviewed by a member of the news team of a Victoria radio station. Among other things, I was asked: "How long have you known that your husband has Hemochromatosis?" and when I replied: "Seven years!" he was visibly taken aback. "Why," he wanted to know, "has it taken you so long to get the society started?"

He is a very nice young man and has been very helpful, but as I didn't have the time or the energy to embark on an explanation which would have required several hours, to say the least, I simply replied: "It took a long time to find enough people . . . !"

The truth was, of course, that ever since Tom was first diagnosed—after years and years of growing progressively worse—and we first heard the unfamiliar term, "Hemochromatosis", we had started immediately, but unsuccessfully, to try to find out more about this disease. We had written dozens of letters hoping that a search would lead us to some sort of association or foundation which we could join, and from which we'd be able to get the information we so desperately needed. The team who were treating him then were simply magnificent and very knowledgeable, but they were always overworked and in too much of a rush to listen to questions which just had to remain unanswered.

We had eagerly absorbed any little snippets of information and, at length, we thought we had learned all there was to know. Only now do we realize how pitifully inadequate that knowledge was. We also realize that there was a great deal we could have been told to reassure us, and, on looking back, we have had to admit that our main source of comfort at that stage sprang from being able to talk to other people who were there receiving treatment at the same time.

It was a happy arrangement that everybody who suffered from Hemochromatosis in that city and surrounding areas, was bled on the same day; at the hematology clinic, by a team of experts.

Blood tests were done early in the morning and everyone sat around anxiously awaiting their results. For new "hemochromatotics" it was a boost when one of the old stagers was told: "You don't have to be bled today. Come back next month" Or, even better: "Come back in three months!" When you are on a twice-a-week schedule—or what M.W. of Terrace aptly describes as "doubles"—it helps to know that it might come to end some time. One day, when Tom was still as brown as a nut and too weak to drive himself home after a phlebotomy, it gave me a tremendous boost when someone said: "I used to be like that two years ago. Just wait. No matter how hopeless it seems now, I promise you it will be better in two years."

That magical phrase... "TWO YEARS!" At times it had seemed like a hundred, but we had clung to that promise like drowning people!

After settling in Calgary, we had continued to investigate the possible existence of a group which we could join, thinking that perhaps we could give similar support to others. If, however, it was a lonely experience to be told that Tom was possibly the only Hemochromatotic under treatment in the city at that time, we could not say that this was a totally unexpected discovery.

We had only to recall the days when Tom was with the airline and how, as our trips internationally had taken us from one city to another, we were distressed to find that in many places so little was known about Hemochromatosis that we had to carry with us a letter of explanation from our own doctor in order to get someone to do a phlebotomy. We had not forgotten that even in Canada we'd invariably had to give our own layman's explanation of what Hemochromatosis is. Leigh's family doctor in Toronto had heard of "Bronze Diabetes" but never thought he'd really see a case and had been genuinely intrigued. When he had agreed to undertake Tom's bleeds each Christmas when we visited Leigh, he had always listened avidly to all we could tell him, for obviously he believed that Tom presented him with a unique opportunity for study.

As my consuming distress about Leigh gave way to fervent gratitude for what she had been spared by timely diagnosis, I became almost frantic to make others aware that Hemochromatosis is primarily an inherited disorder; *other families had to know! I could not accept that so few were afflicted; but even if there was only one, he or she had to be contacted!*

For all I knew, that person, whoever he or she might be, had been fortunate enough to find a competent physician who would take the necessary steps. Our experience had taught me, however, that there were not many doctors who screened relatives, and very few would have requisitioned iron overload tests for a woman as young as Leigh.

At first I tried to evade what was obviously my responsibility. My own life was far from easy at the time. I worked long hours and saw little enough of my family as it was. I did not know the laws of Canada; I did not know where to begin; I had no money. But, at last, I faced it. It was no use waiting around for "someone to do something about it!" If anyone was going to set the ball rolling to give Hemochromatosis a higher profile and stimulate some public awareness, it was going to have to be me.

It was not long before I had to admit to myself that I could achieve nothing on my own. How could one start a society without members? Tom, Leigh and I hardly represented a forceful body. Besides, I needed to learn more about other people's experiences and I had to raise money somehow for registration, and other expenses.

I had once thought and hoped that publication in a magazine with wide circulation would bring me into contact with people with similar problems. For months and months I had laboured over an article. I had described, graphically, the agony Tom had endured during the five years in which he grew sicker and sicker until he was close to death, because no doctor could diagnose the true cause of his suffering. I had told of the miracle that had finally led him to someone who recognized the symptoms of Hemochromatosis. When one editor was not interested, I tried another. It became increasingly clear that my story would be more credible if I could give other case histories to support our story. Whenever a magazine informed me that my article was good and made interesting reading, there was the inevitable backing off: a doctor on their advisory panel was of the opinion that the disease was far too rare to be of interest to the public. The observation that continued to rankle the most, was the one that Tom's experience was unfortunate but we were really to blame for not having gone to the right doctors in the first place!. . . . How I wish that I could get that editor and his staff doctor to read some of the letters that have since been written to me by others, describing experiences that precisely parallel ours! Years and years of sickness, going from doctor to doctor before diagnosis; destruction of body—and sometimes mind—and the tragic impairment of the quality of life.

But in 1982, it all still seemed a "catch 22" situation. I needed to get the story into print in order to reach others who would substantiate what I said; I had to make contact with Hemochromatosis victims in order to get a society off the ground, but no publication would help me in my search until I could prove that Tom and Leigh were not unique. Meanwhile, I had been reading enough medical literature to make me realize how many people were at risk and I was making myself literally sick with the urgency of it all. Oh, the frustration! If only all phlebotomies were carried out at a central treatment centre I would have found some of the people who later joined us, much sooner. What an opportunity I had let slip when I could have taken the names and addresses of the people at that first hemotology clinic in Johannesburg!

So much research had and was being done. If I, a lay person, could obtain and read what these wonderful researchers had written, why couldn't every physician—especially family doctors? The public had to be told and we needed people to join us in our campaign. The medical profession had to be prodded to be on the lookout for what might be right under their noses.

About this time Tom and Leigh were coming home from their phlebotomies at the Ambulatory Daycare Unit of the Victoria General Hospital with the interesting information that—although it was not a special clinic where all hemochromatotics, specifically, were treated, and even then not simultaneously—others were being bled there. With each report my excitement grew.

Right here, on my own doorstep, so to speak, there might be enough people at least to attend an inaugural meeting—but the medical profession are ethically prevented from disclosing the names of their patients and, in any case, I did not know which doctors, apart from our family doctor and the specialist who was then treating Tom and Leigh, had hemochromatotic patients.

As I could not lie in wait for people as they emerged from the daycare unit, I tried to enlist the aid of the medical reporter of the Times-Colonist in Victoria. Unfortunately I failed to convince him that Hemochromatosis was of sufficient interest to warrant a column which might urge people to get into touch with me; consequently the sympathetic ear given me by Sheryl Craig-Merrett, at the rooms of Leigh's and Tom's specialist, was a welcome change.

Naturally she could not disclose to me the names of any patients, but she promised that she would tell them about me and she gave me a list of hematologists at universities and major hospitals in Montreal, Toronto, Calgary, New Westminster and Vancouver, to whom I could write.

Many, many hours of letter-writing ensued and I just couldn't wait for the replies. I haunted the mailbox and it seemed that I waited an eternity. In one sense, when they did arrive, the responses were terribly disappointing, for these specialists could give me no statistics whatsoever, and not one of them had had a patient for some time, but the letters were kind and encouraging and, in time, would teach me a very valuable lesson.

My immediate reaction was one of astonishment. Was it possible that in a small city like Victoria, there were several people who suffered from Hemochromatosis, while in those major centres these eminent physicians were not currently treating a single patient? Either the doctors in Victoria were brighter than elsewhere in Canada, I told myself, or, having become aware of the incidence of Hemochromatosis, they were on the lookout for and consequently diagnosing more people. How could I seek out those patients?

I know now that all phlebotomies are not performed by Hematologists and that I should have written to a wider spectrum of specialists from Gastro-enterologists to Rheumatologists.

The first break came when I began to give organ lessons to Agnes Schuitema whose husband, Reindeer, is the host of a very popular garden programme on CFMS radio. They both proved to be good friends and really encouraged me. They were sufficiently sympathetic for Reindeer to slip an appeal into his Sunday morning programme which is heard over a wide area. Almost simultaneously, Leigh and Tom found another good friend in Dorothy Found of the Ambulatory Day Care Unit. Dorothy undertook to tell patients about the proposed society and to direct them to where they could find us if they wished to do so.

What an exciting day it was when Don Taylor first walked into the piano and organ store where Tom and I were working and said: "Dorothy sent me to you. I have Hemochromatosis!"

It was five years since Tom had been able to compare notes with anyone. I guess Don had never had the opportunity to do so; and the two of them nearly talked their heads off. It was the same, a few days later, when Bill R. and Roy McLeod came along. My pen absolutely flew as I tried to record what they were telling us, for their symptoms were so different from what Tom had experienced, and they were not even particularly brown (although Don Taylor's hands are very deeply pigmented and Tom Rogerson, whose acquaintance we made shortly after this, has the familiar "tan"). Denise Wiggins was the first lady to seek us out and we were thrilled to meet her.

The night before Patty Pitts and her Chek Television crew were due to interview us, we held our first meeting. It took place in our home and I arrived from work just as Don and Roy were crossing the street from where they had parked their cars. I watched them as they approached and I recognized them by the way they walked; slowly, painfully, the way Tom does, because their bones hurt. (I was astounded to learn later from Maureen Worobey that she has had stiff joints since she was only twenty-one!)

That meeting greatly increased my self-confidence and determination. Despite years of training in public speaking and public relations, I am a self-confessed moral coward when I am personally involved, but I was now speaking on behalf of others. I had been put down as a sentimentalist prone to melodrama and generalization, but now I had proof that others had been through as gruelling a time as Tom had, before diagnosis, and I knew that many others would suffer similarly unless increased public awareness led to *their* diagnosis. I kept that thought with me throughout the first television interview and again on the Ida Clarkson Show. I was subsequently interviewed twice on CBC, the Vancouver Sun ran an excellent article and we appeared on the BCTV News, which brought more letters and phone calls.

I wept over some of those letters. Imagine the agony, mental as well a physical, of a young man in his mid thirties with his pancreas destroyed and "only half a liver"! Picture the bewilderment of a young wife whose husband has had to tell her that their sex-life is virtually at an end! What do I say to a girl in her early thirties who had not menstruated for more than two years and wonders whether this is due to the phlebotomies. Will she ever have a child, she asks me. How should I know? I wish I did—but I'm not a doctor.

I vowed that I would try to read all that had ever been written on the subject and I would find doctors who could give us the answers we all so desperately needed. Somehow we would prove that Hemochromatosis was not as rare as was generally believed, and that the statistics were out of date; we'd strive to find those who were at risk *before* the damage was done.

To the Hampton family of Terrace, B.C., and this includes

Maureen Worobey, who was a Hampton before her marriage, I owe more than I can say. They have taught me so much. When I first wrote to them asking for information, the response was spontaneous and whole-hearted. They could have ignored me or told me to mind my own business. Instead they embraced the cause along with me.

I have their snapshots beside me as I write this, and regard them now as family. Maureen's son, Todd, was until recently, the youngest subscribing member of this society. She, Maureen, writes enthusiastic and newsy letters and she is the representative of the society in that part of the world. Jorunn is the wife of Gary Hampton, Maureen's brother, and I am indebted to Jorunn for her long, informative letter. Right from the start they have all been so supportive that I used to send them tapes of radio and television interviews, as a sort of up-date on progress, and I was so happy when I could finally send them the minutes of our inaugural meeting in Victoria. What I was especially grateful for, however, was their immediate consent to the use of their names and case histories whenever and wherever this should prove necessary. My greatest obstacle, all along, lay in trying to convince those who most needed convincing that the experience of my own family was not unique, and the Hampton's story supports this. Some doctors are affronted when I say that Hemochromatosis is a "little-known disease." The ones who take exception—and who could blame them?—are those who *are* familiar with the condition. Every second letter I receive, however, only serves to emphasize how rare such doctors are, and those who were guided to them at the outset are more fortunate than they realize.

Until I read Maureen's letter, I had thought Leigh, my daughter, to be about the youngest person ever to have such a massive iron-overload. I had been told that women were not at risk—and if they were, it would only be after menopause—and here was Maureen offering further evidence to disprove this. Men were at risk but would manifest the symptoms in their middle years—yet here was Gary, in his thirties with Hemochromatosis almost as far advanced as my husband's had been at fifty!

In 1981 I had received a letter from Doctor S.C. Naiman of the Vancouver General Hospital in which he mentioned a young woman in her early 30's with primary Hemochromatosis, but at that stage something else in the letter had made more of an impact than the youthful age of the patient. What had really riveted my attention was the sentence in which Doctor Naiman explained that the young lady in question was "the daughter of a known patient who was a carrier of Hemochromatosis." A *carrier*? I had never heard of this before. Could people pass on the gene to others and yet not suffer the involvements of the disease themselves? This was indeed food for thought.

Maureen's first letter came while I was still wondering about this. I quote from her letter.

"Our whole family and spouses*(mine will be checked this trip down) have seen and given blood to Dr. P. MacLeod of the New Grace Hospital at Shaughnessy so they have a file on us. My older sister was found to be a carrier but will not have any problems from it. All spouses are clear so the second generation will not suffer from it but they do carry the mutant gene; so when they marry the intended wife or husband should check to see if things will go wrong again.

"I have an appointment on August 11 at the Genetics Unit to see Doctor Judith Allanson, who has taken over Dr. MacLeod's cases. My husband will be checked and I will give them any new information they require."

Maureen set me wondering about myself. Was it true that both parents would have to carry the gene before a child would develop the complications of primary Hemochromatosis? All my previous assertions were now questionable. I was shaken. If Leigh was unable to reject excess iron, I could no longer simply assume that she'd inherited this from her father. I, too, must carry a gene. And since Tom had Hemochromatosis to such a severe degree, it was not sufficient to ascribe this to a gene he'd inherited from his father alone. What about his mother's family? What about mine?

* On their way down to Vancouver, the Worobeys were involved in a car accident in which her husband was killed.

CHAPTER TWO

BY THE EARLY PART OF 1983, WE HAD MEMBERS AS FAR afield as Ontario and Washington State. I took a trip which brought dozens of inquires from Calgary. I envisaged a branch there and another in Edmonton.

Letters continued to pour in:

"Dear Mrs. Warder,

I've been thinking about you a lot lately and wondering if everything is going all right, first with your husband and daughter & with the Association & all the members out there. . . I'd really like to hear from fellow sufferers. However, maybe everyone is too tired to write. I see by one of your letters that your husband gets severely tired spells, so that must be one of the conditions we can't seem to cure. I only know how exhausted I feel most of the time, ability to exert getting less; getting to be an awful effort to get up and move at all. Plus now very sore ankle and feet tendons & joints. That's no help. . . Well, I went in April for my 2nd liver biopsy & was found very low in iron (deficient in fact). They didn't find cirrhosis & they can't do tests to assess any permanent damage in other organs. My heart feels the most tired. I'm on Digoxin, also Prednisone for pituitary. Next they think I'm getting an enlarged thyroid, so I'm on thyroid pills since a month. It's quite a battle & I don't envy a Dr's dilemmas. I find the hot humid weather quite unbearable & have to stay indoors in an airconditioned room a lot of the time. . . I do not talk about my symptoms or feelings to anyone, as there's no way to make any-

one understand & everyone else has his or her own problems. . . . I do hope you are well yourself & everyone still able to cope with all the problems.''   E.C. , Ontario
(Many others reported that they could not stand heat).

"I enjoyed hearing from you. Use my name if any help. . . . My writing has also been affected. I have no strength in my hands—hence the unsteady writing.'' M. Duck, Prince George (Since deceased. Her death was a sad blow as she became a good friend and a loyal supporter of the C H S).

"My husband has had this disease, which was diagnosed in Toronto, since 1970. Until we moved to Calgary from Northern Ontario in 1977, he had no problems having blood removed regularly. But until the end of 1982, when he got in touch with a new doctor, he had a lot of problems as they didn't seem to understand Hemochromatosis and consequently did not feel the iron & other levels tied in,. . . or that the procedure which had been recommended by a specialist, should be followed.

We don't fully understand the problem and would like more information. We wish we could have seen you or heard you speak on the subject. We would appreciate any information you would have, that you could send us.''   J.P., Alberta

"We recently read an article in the Calgary Herald daily newspaper (April 26/83—copy enclosed) which is of great interest to me. My husband is currently being investigated for hemochromatosis—having been in hospital for one month during January for swelling of ankles and legs. For years he has been treated for high blood pressure and a chronic back condition (herniated discs). However, while in hospital he was quite jaundiced and they discovered iron overload. He presently has blood taken once every three weeks at a specialty clinic of Calgary General Hospital. The jaundice is still apparent but not to the extent it was in January. Our specialist is placing him on a salt restricted diet—low protein—and increasing carbohydrates.

"His blood has become very thin and they are very much afraid of any bleeding. So much so, that they are unable to do an ordinary liver biopsy. However, they hope to obtain a device from Montreal to do a biopsy by putting a tube down a vein (or artery) to the liver. His swelling has decreased considerably but his circulation is not too good. There is still some swelling in the liver area. Prior to being diagnosed as above, he did have very dark ankles and backs of his hands (were dark)—however, we did not suspect this to be abnormal as during the summer months these parts of his body were exposed to the sun. The heart specialist that he attended for high blood pressure just assumed that the ankles were dark from periodic swelling and put this down to water retention.

Any information you can send to me would be very much appreciated. My husband does not recall any problem in his family (father or mother both deceased). The article mentioned symptoms such as fatigue, dizziness and loss of memory. My husband suffers fatigue only—no dizziness or loss of memory. Thank you for your interest and concern." H.D., Calgary (Husband died after massive hemorrhage from throat).

"My case was diagnosed last July, However, out of all the blood tests I only had a trace of sugar in two. I have never been bronze coloured. My family, that have been tested, do *not* have the disease.

I had approximately 35 phlebotomies or blood lettings. I have never had loss of memory. They took 500 ccs. twice a week for the first two months, then once a week until my iron test was normal. I make sure I get less than 5 grams of iron a day and will keep getting blood tests.

I have had over 30 transfusions, so this could have been part of it." D.C., Calgary

"I have just read your article in the Calgary "Herald" concerning Hemochromatosis. I am curious to know, how a Dr. determines whether a person has hemochromatosis. Any information you can supply would be greatly appreciated."

Mrs. C.M., Calgary

"Could you please send me information on Hemochromatosis as per your article in the Calgary Herald. My father died of this disease and our family was told it was brought on by drinking too much beer. I would like to have further information regarding this killer." C.L.W., Calgary (Could be the doctors were right. But there are an awful lot of Mormons in Salt Lake City who have Hemochromatosis and have never touched a drop of liquor in their lives. Someone else had been told a similar story and, when tested, appeared to have inherited HH from the undiagnosed parent!)

CHAPTER THREE

BY NOW, OF COURSE, I HAD REALIZED THAT HEMOCHROMA-
tosis (HH) was not just the medical term for "Bronze Diabetes"
or "Pigmented Cirrhosis". There are many facets of the disease
and many victims are neither bronzed nor diabetic. I had read a
great deal, but from Don Taylor, Tom Rogerson (who became
the first national chairman) and from Roy McLeod of Victoria, as
well as from the Hamptons, I learned first-hand that arthritis is a
common complaint; that periods of dreadful fatigue are experienced by all. It was B.C. of Guelph who first made me wonder
how HH could be misdiagnosed as Lupus.

Roy McLeod was the first person I had actually met who
suspected that his iron overload had been induced—which meant
that his condition was not hereditary; in other words it was not
primary Hemochromatosis. It was to transpire years later—by
which time he would be virtually handicapped as a result of the
crippling effects of excess iron—that he was, in fact, a carrier of
a single gene.

At that stage, in my early groping for information and thirst for
knowledge, it was a particularly sad disappointment to learn that
the famous Professor Clement Finch whose name, like that of
T.H. Bothwell, was, to me, synonymous with research into the
consequences of iron overload, had been in Victoria and I had
missed meeting him. I wrote to him and was honoured to receive
not only a prompt reply but copies of one of his most recent
papers. I must have read and re-read it a hundred times. Then,

with the assistance of my good friend, Johann van Reenen, chief librarian of the Victoria Medical and Hospital Libraries for the Greater Victoria Hospital Society, references which appeared at the end of the publication became the springboard for further study.

And as I read more and more, in the face of the tragic experiences which afflicted people were pouring out to me, I was obsessed by what I could only regard as a tragedy. Researchers could devote their lives to probing the mysteries of life and death, they could offer the key to improved health and prolonged life, but there was no way in which they could force the average practising physician to grasp that key. The deeper I delved, the more overwhelmed I became; by all that was there to be learned, on the one hand, and by the cruel consequences of delayed diagnosis, on the other. . . . all because, to too many members of the medical profession, Hemochromatosis remained only ''a question in an examination paper''.

Inevitably, whenever I appeared on a radio or television program, the interview with me would be followed by a discussion with someone estimated to be really knowlegeable; and the expert would then thoroughly discredit me by insisting that, at most, one person in twenty thousand was at risk. One Toronto authority went as far as to suggest one in a hundred thousand.

I could not have continued if my family had not been so wonderfully supportive. A very large proportion of my earnings was being poured into the expenses of a growing project and when I was short of postage or couldn't pay the exhorbitant phone bill, I borrowed from Tom. He ''lent'' me the money without expecting to be paid back. Leigh did most of the legwork involved in the registration. She also helped with typing and did all the artwork for the newsletter. Shaun began work on a data base, staying up far into the night to write the programs and Deborah, our dear, newly-acquired daughter-in-law,took over as ''girl friday'', even to the extent of producing our letterheads. She used Leigh's design for the logo, while Tom provided the lettering; painstakingly done with aching hands.

My grandchildren willingly did their share, friends helped in the most wonderful way and even my customers and music pupils at the store were swept up in the activity.

With their help the first "music swapathon" was launched to raise funds. Victoria's musicians were encouraged to bring along an unwanted music book or piece of sheet music and fifty cents, and they were then permitted to exchange what they had brought, for whatever took their fancy. As some people simply donated music without dipping into the bin for something else, we soon had a good selection for the choosing and our swapathon, which fortunately enjoyed the blessing of my employers and the mall management, became quite an institution.

In order to keep the "Hemie" funds—as they soon became known—separate from the store revenue, we made a cash box out of a large carton and labelled it in big letters : IN AID OF THE CANADIAN HEMOCHROMATOSIS SOCIETY.

One Saturday, just before closing time, a middle-aged man came to the counter to pay for a store purchase. My trusty volunteers had gone home for the day, leaving the "Hemie" box beside me for safe-keeping. They placed it in such a way that the gentleman was obliged to read the writing on it, upside down.

He stood for some moments, peering at the lettering, twisting his head and obviously intrigued by what he read there. I studied his bent head, fascinated for reasons of my own. Had I not seen hair like that before. . . . ?

In less than a second I went on an incredible journey. . . . **seventeen thousand miles. . . . thirty five years. . . . !**

. . . . There was nothing fluttery about Tom's mother, I observed at our first meeting. Later, looking at snapshots of her standing next to a nineteen year-old Tom—he with his arm around her shoulders and she gazing up with a doting expression at her Herculean son—I was surprised to see how small she really was, for she gave the impression of being taller and, somehow more robust. Her menfolk adored her and, especially because I knew nothing about mothers of boys and had never met anyone quite like her, she intrigued me; "one of the guys", with a weakness for frothy, lace frills at the throat and wrists, and stylish little hats with sleek, shiny feathers. She had started out as a first-class classical violinist. When I met her she could swing it with the best. The only time she ever sulked was if Pop dared to tell her she'd played a wrong note.

I concluded that, if my mother were inclined to primness, it was because she only had daughters. Raised under a petticoat government, my conversation was peppered with euphemisms. I had never been permitted to say "stink". None of us would use "lie" if "fib" would do. Tom and Selby, on the other hand, could say the most outrageous things in front of **their** mother who, while she tolerated no disrespect or vulgarity, would simply double up with mirth and laugh until she coughed. The secret must lie, I decided with the wisdom of seventeen years, in the fact that her household was predominantly male.

She chain-smoked, and to this I attributed the colour of her skin and the myriads of lines which creased her face. Although she could not have been more then forty-four at the time, she seemed old to me. Women generally appeared to be older for their years then, than they do today—or it could just have been that I was so young. But she did look old; and yet her hair was like a child's. My mum, whose entire family were magnificently and prematurely grey, envied Rae her light-brown, baby-fine hair without a trace of silver in it.

. . . . **The man before me had identical hair. It wasn't really light-brown after all; more a light, no-colour. . . . And I'd since encountered a number of people with hair like that. . . . What about Tom's? . . . .**

. . . . On weekdays during the war, while Tom was away at the air force camp, I would contrive all manner of errands and invent lame excuses for visiting his parents. There were photographs on their walls at which one could steal surreptitious glances if they were present, or gaze longingly when they were out of the room.

A shortage of fuel and tyres had long since reduced me to going everywhere on foot and, as I went about the business of gathering news for my paper, it was simple to make a short detour and drop in, even during working hours for a quick cup of tea. Frequently I would find Tom's mother lying down. She would call out at my knock and, hearing my voice, invite me to let myself in. "Feeling 'fluey' again," she would inevitably explain, with an apologetic smile, and struggle up, smoothing her hair and looking altogether different from the cheerful "good chum" image she presented when her menfolk were around.

. . . . I stood in that store on that Saturday afternoon and writhed in mental agony. I recalled every detail of Rae's agonizing death and wept inside for her ravaged beautiful son. . . .

My customer looked up, smiling quizzically; eyes still narrowed from trying to decipher words from the wrong angle. His face was nutbrown, deeply wrinkled and his chest and arms were practically hairless.

"Couldn't believe my eyes," he said. " A society for HEMOCHROMATOSIS!. . . Until this moment I believed that I was about the only person in the world who had it!"

Before long it seemed that I had no life at all beyond my job and the society. Businesses in shopping malls are dictated to by the owners of those malls and, as the hours of operation were progressively extended, I was frequently required to work 65 hours or more a week. When I arrived home at night, it was either to find a pile of correspondence waiting for me, or the red light on the answering machine to rivet my attention as I walked in at the door. I thought longingly of the days when I had taught school and wondered why I had ever thought a school day too long.

The **Hammy** became my mobile office. It was parked near the store so that I could catch up on correspondence during my very infrequent coffee or lunchbreak; rare days off were taken up in the same way. I wrote letters in the car; I wrote letters in restaurants and while waiting for a doctor or a dentist. Because I was so tired, I was chronically nauseous; and because the tragic stories which had been relayed to me over the telephone in my absence, upset me so much that I couldn't sleep, we reached a stage where Tom put his foot down and forbade me to play back messages on the answering machine before I went to bed.

On Tuesdays I taught organ lessons on Saltspring Island and as Tom took me there in the **Hammy**, the work went on while we travelled to and fro on the ferry—as it did during periodic visits to Vancouver to be with Shaun and Deborah. I scribbled under the dryer at the hairdresser's and feverishly made notes. My mind swam with information, for in addition to the daily correspondence and research required for the articles I kept sending to newspapers and periodicals, I had now been confronted with the unexpected.

On the night before the application for the incorporation of the society was submitted to the Registrar, I had lain awake half the night in a cold sweat. I had realized, almost in terror, that my life might never be the same again. I would be plunged into everything that such an undertaking entailed. . . . annual general meetings!. . . . minutes!. . . . financial statements. . . . ! Optimism had finally prevailed, however. There did not have to be a lifetime of commitment. Someone, somewhere in some pie-in-the-sky place, would come forward with the know-how, and in some miraculous way take over in due course. By focusing attention on the situation, we would have provided the catalyst; there would be a chain-reaction of an equally miraculous nature. Soon doctors everywhere would be so clued-up and take such good care of their hemochromatotic patients that the society would become redundant. Of course the Government of Canada would by this time have made it mandatory for iron supplements to carry a warning label—so providing an example which goverments throughout the world would be swift to follow—and a blood test for iron overload would have become routine; particularly for diabetics and arthritics.

As I pinned my faith on what the medical profession would do FOR me, I never for one moment dreamed that any physician would, in turn, ever require anything **of** me. . . . !

Until one day a request arrived in the mail, from a doctor in Calgary. . . . '' Please send me a supply of patient literature and any other information you have available.''

''My doctor advised me to contact you,'' wrote a lady from Hamilton, Ontario, two days later.

This was a development for which I had not bargained. I tried to deal with it immediately, but, quite understandably, not one of the many, knowledgeable, busy specialists whom I approached was inclined to take time out to provide the copy for such a brochure. The last one I went to see was a geneticist, and I'm glad I did. I am truly indebted to him for the kind and patient manner in which he answered my questions for, until then, the genetics of HH was the one aspect I had found most difficult to grasp in the course of my ''home study course''. I was also excited to be told again by him of the work being done at Grace Hospital in Vancouver by people like Dr. Judith Allanson. I wrote to her and, in due course, she consented to becoming one of our first honorary medical directors.

But the geneticist did not volunteer to write a brochure for me.

When I very diffidently broached the subject of "patient" material, his response, while gratifying in one respect, was hardly comforting. "Mrs. Warder," he said, " you probably know as much about Hemochromatosis as anyone on this island."

He advised me to try the "March of Dimes"—which had sponsored information on other diseases—and gave me a printed list of names and addresses of geneticists who possibly carried out genetic (HLA) tissue typing in Canada, for which I was grateful. At the same time he cautioned that I might not get too far in that direction either. Most genetic researchers and specialists, he told me, are more involved with pediatric disorders than those which genetically afflict adults.

It was a good thing that I proceeded to wear metaphorical blinkers. If I had known then that two years down the road, despite a program of fanatical dedication which would almost destroy Tom, demand total commitment of my family and impair my own health, I would still be told by the Executive Director of a prominent Canadian health foundation: "You'll never get anywhere with this. Hemochromatosis is not a marketable commodity!" my resolve might have wavered. My optimism would certainly have worn thin.

The mail brought one request after another. There was no escape. I would have to write my own "patient literature". Fortunately there was a reprieve. While I was still labouring over the copy for the brochure, we had a lucky break. Dennis Elsom, publisher of the North Delta Sentinel gave us a generous supply of reprints of an article he had agreed to publish in his newspaper, and for some months we were able to comply with requests for literature by mailing these as a stop-gap. Reading one of those pamphlets today, I am amazed at how much more has been written on the subject since then, what strides have been made in research and how much greater the awareness of HH is today. I am astounded—most particularly—at how unbelievably the estimates for incidence have risen.

How grateful I suddenly was, for the invaluable experience gained years before when I worked for the phamaceutical company. With Deborah able to produce it in the right format, we finally brought out a brochure and the Canadian Hemochromatosis Society was able to provide the first—and, for several years, the only—"patient information" on Hemochromatosis, readily available to the Canadian public. And such is the nature of Canada's people, that a diagnosis of an HH victim somewhere on one side of the country, frequently meant alerting and monitoring relatives at the opposite end of the continent—or even overseas. It was not long before our little green booklets were travelling around the world.

We were making progress but I was exhausted. One day Tom made a decision. Out of the blue we had found a buyer for our house, which meant that we were now in a position to move to the mainland. Vancouver was considered more accessible to our members, two of our honorary directors and medical advisers were at UBC and if he, Tom, returned to the job he had held when we had lived in the **Hammy**, I would be able to stay home for a while, regain my health and promote the society.

Before we left Victoria, the "island branch" of the family—consisting of Tom and me, our son-in-law, Bruce, our two rather apprehensive grandchildren and Leigh—went along to the city's excellent new hospital where we all had blood taken for HLA (genetic) tissue typing and for a complete iron profile. Shaun and Deborah had their tests done at Vancouver General Hospital on the same day, to make the family study complete.

Before I fell asleep that night, I thought with gratitude of all the work which must have been done by researchers for them to have come up with the necessary diagnostic tools to make the future safe for Tom's and my descendants, and I hoped a day would come when all relatives of known victims would be similarly screened. Which is why today our society leaves no stone unturned to try and achieve this. Which is why we have made our motto: "Find us one afflicted person and we have hope of saving an entire family!"

CHAPTER FOUR

IT WAS PROFESSOR FINCH WHO WROTE TO TELL ME OF THE existence of the newly-established Hemochromatosis Research Foundation in Albany, New York. I lost no time in writing to the founder, Dr. Margit Krikker; an eminently suitable person to head up such an organization as her husband had died of Hemochromatosis. She seemed equally pleased to learn of our society, telephoned in response to my communication and followed this up with a letter.

She wrote: "As there is strength in numbers, and knowledge is gained from exchange of ideas, I hope that, as you suggested, we can and will co-operate with each other, and achieve our common goals: to find and prophylactically bleed the young hemochromatotic and prevent the lethal complications; find and treat the older hemochromatotic and reverse his complications, obtain funds for prevalence studies and necessary research, and eventually be able to assist families of hemochromatotics financially."

Since then she has repeatedly proved to be a very present help in time of trouble, particularly when I have been at my wits end as to what was best for Tom.

Here was a woman after my own heart—and a doctor to boot! She endeared herself to me by her remark: "And they would have us believe that it (HH) is a rare bird!"

Just before talking to her, I had written to a doctor at Vancouver General Hospital, explaining that I wanted to know more about HH for an article I was writing. His reply had been prompt and very kind, but had concluded with: "Because of the rarity of the disorder, I am uncertain as to whether there would be wide-spread interest in this condition; but, nevertheless, if you would approach the article more on the basis of living with a chronic disease which is of genetic origin this would probably have much more widespread interest."

This despite the fact that, some years before that, Corwin Q. Edwards et al had written in the New England Journal of Medicine, July 7, 1977, "The frequency of Hemochromatosis in the population is unquestionably underestimated."

And now here was Dr. Krikker telling me that an estimated 10-13% of the population were carriers of one gene for HH and that 1 in 333 were at risk of developing the full-blown disease![(ii)]From her we learned that a protocol was under review by the Institute Review Board of the Albany Medical College and, as soon as it had been approved, the Hemochromatosis Research Institute would be assisted by the American Red Cross in the screening of all blood donors in the Albany area of the state of New York. In this important, pilot program, transferrin saturation of 55% and over would be the test to determine potential Hemochromatosis.

Spurred on by this, Shaun and I embarked, in 1983, on what was, for us, a monumental undertaking; an attempt to create nation-wide awareness among physicians in Canada. We wanted a large-scale program for checking Canadians, too, and were de-termined, furthermore, to establish a central registry of all known victims, which would enable us to monitor families. As a start, letters were written to the registrars of medical bodies throughout the country, advising them of the existence of the society and what had been accomplished; outlining what we hoped to achieve and pleading for their co-operation. Replies were received from all provinces and territories, with the exception of Alberta and Saskatchewan; the Manitobans requiring further evidence of our credibility.

The "campaign", which went on for six months involved a tremendous amount of work. Since, in many cases, information concerning the society was forwarded by the recipient of our first letter, to other members of these associations, a second, and sometimes a third letter had to be written in reply to theirs. We could never have coped without Deborah and our volunteer secretary, Marianne Green. The results made us very hopeful.

Naturally, we received many letters in which their writers expressed sentiments ranging from scepticism to outright scorn. Some doctors, as we anticipated, told us the old, old story. . . . they had never seen a case of HH and doubted that they ever would; others, quite understandably, wished to know more about the aims of the society and our credibility before committing themselves. However, there were sufficient expressions of genuine interest and offers of help—at the **specialist level**-- to reward our efforts, and we felt like framing the half-page notice which appeared in the Quebec Medical journal, BULLETIN.

Unfortunately we had to concede that our efforts had gone nowhere spectacular as far as the **family** physician was concerned. This was the area we deemed most critical.

Despite some element of disillusionment, however, our so-called "awareness campaign" turned out to be an invaluable, personal experience. As I later wrote, I had hitherto divided members of the medical profession into three, distinct categories and my opinion of them varied accordingly: for the researcher, admiration which bordered on hero-worship; profound respect for the doctor who knew about Hemochromatosis; contempt for the one who did not. It was shattering to realize that there were doctors who, themselves, had suffered the ravages of HH and were interested in joining the society. They, too, had become the victims of delayed diagnosis and treatment; not because their colleagues were guilty of neglect or malpractice. . . . solely because the belief persisted that HH was rare. A physician, rushed off his feet in a busy practice, can hardly be blamed for not devoting hours to the study of a disease of which few medical dictionaries even give mention! No wonder he doesn't recognize it when he sees it!

Hardly a day went by without someone asking for more information than a brochure, by nature of its size, could provide. Unfortunately we were desperately short of funds.

As the work we did was too wide in scope and did not tie in with the general, bureacratic definition of "research"—and also because HH was considered unworthy of interest—we did not qualify for government assistance. I tried the United Way but it was obvious that, the instant I brought "iron overload" into the conversation, I had blown it. Doesn't EVERYONE KNOW that one cannot have too much iron? I was not even put through to the person whom I was calling.

There was only one way in which we could hope to answer most of the questions with which we were bombarded and, at the same time, pass on some of the personal experiences which so many victims of Hemochromatosis had shared with me. Tom had bought us a computer and and printer at the time we started setting up the registry and data base, and Shaun had risked both mind and soul, if not life and limb, in initiating his mother into the terrible, awesome world of high tech.

Many nights, after I had spent the day at the computer, I was unable to sleep. I hated what I was doing. But Shaun was a relentless taskmaster and, with Leigh to do the graphics, Deb the format, and Tom financing us, we produced the booklet: "Iron— the other side of the story!" Made up of extracts from my book, it remains to this day, the society's only ongoing source of income. We concluded with an extract from a letter written to me by a prominent Canadian surgeon, in which he decribed what he had suffered. It told of how a brilliant career had been cut short by crippling joint disease. . . . caused by Hemochromatosis.

How thrilled we were when, among the first orders received, there were over twenty from doctors! The knowledge that every one of them was an expert on HH, filled me with trepidation; which is to be expected, I guess, when the amateur subjects his or her work to the scrutiny of the professional.

As soon as the "booklet" was ready—as had been the case when we produced the brochure— copies were sent to members of our family in several countries. One of the books went to a cousin who is a doctor of some repute. The information elicited little or no response, and I could relate to those who complained that they had tried in vain to alert relatives to the dangers of untreated HH. There is always an element of shock; sometimes perhaps suspicion; some people are affronted or ashamed at being told that they may have inherited a genetic disorder. There is a prevailing "ostrich with its head in the sand" syndrome which I soon learned to expect. But I found, too, that, around the world there were physicians who either refused to order the necessary tests or were ignorant as to what form such tests should take.

My sister— one of my few relatives who did request that she be checked—was told that results could only be obtained by processing her blood in the United States. It was to be expected that, when Tom's brother assured us that he and his daughter had been found to be "not at risk", I could not help doubting what I had heard. I had learned from experience that, internationally, family doctors in general still applied the same test for iron overload as they did for iron deficiency; mistakenly especting that hemoglobin levels would be elevated, whereas, in HH, they are normal.

All of us would have to try harder. In our Spring/Summer 1984 newsletter, we were happy to report:
"We are pleased to inform you that this society has become an affiliate of the Hemochromatosis Research Foundation. Since October 13, 1983, together with Sweden, Germany, Mexico and Luxembourg, we form part of what shows every sign of becoming an international research foundation. This organization is, of course, a professional body, while ours is a 'patient' or grass roots society."

In the same newsletter I confessed: "The letters which we have received from doctors who, themselves, are afflicted with HH, have left me deeply ashamed and contrite. Too often I have accused the physicians, in my mind, of downright ignorance and carelessness in permitting Hemochromatosis to devastate my family in the way it did. I blamed the doctor and not the IRON for what it has done to us—and to you. It has been a humbling and worthwhile lesson to discover how many medical men have suffered as long as some of you before the correct diagnosis was made, and how many failed to detect what now seem like such very obvious signs in their own wives and families. These are among the people who have promised us their help, and together we are going to work towards a common goal: increased public awareness and—most important of all—the heightened awareness of the practising physician.

As I wrote this, I hoped fervently that there would some day be a professional branch of the Canadian Hemochromatosis Society, but that would take another four years.

By December, 1984, we were working steadily on our data base and bulletin board. The central registry of HH sufferers was growing by the day. A television program featuring a member from Port Coquitlam, as well as an article in the Vancouver Sun brought a spate of new diagnoses. As we had anticipated, family members had to be alerted—despite the fact that some of them lived as far away as France and Great Britain. It was gratifying to receive a request for information on iron-overload from a scientist in England.

We shall always be grateful to Doctor Zelig Hurwitz, not only for having been instrumental in Leigh's diagnosis, but for agreeing to become one of the society's first Honorary Directors. It is also a continuing source of gratitude to me that Doctor Robert Raine, a Victoria Gastroenterologist, was willing—at that early stage— to join Doctors Hurwitz and Allanson on the Board, so lending credibility to what could otherwise have become no more than a support group. When Doctor Allanson moved to Arizona, she (reminding us that most geneticists were more involved in pediatric genetics than they were in genetic disorders which afflict adults) advised us to try and persuade a physician of whom she thought very highly, to take her place. We accordingly, and with some diffidence, approached Doctor Michael Hayden, Associate Professor of Medical Genetics and Internal Medicine, and the Director of the Adult Genetics Clinic at the University of British Columbia. We were quite overwhelmed when he consented. He agreed, in addition, to becoming one of the medical advisers to the society.

In due course we were proud not only to add to our Board of Directors as well as to our Advisory Board, the name of Doctor Urs Steinbrecher, Assistant Professor of Medicine, Division of Gastroenterology at UBC, but were able to announce that Doctor Leslie Valberg—now Dean of Medicine at the University of Western Ontario, and known world-wide as a prominent researcher and authority on the treatment of HH—would act as the chief medical adviser to the society. The role played by all these eminent gentlemen in heightening awareness of Hemochromatosis and in assisting us to carry on the work of the Canadian Hemochromatosis Society has been of immeasurable value.

When Tom and I had moved from Victoria to the mainland, we had been obliged to leave behind us not only Leigh and her family but some of our other, dedicated helpers. Fortunately, with the assistance of the Richmond Volunteer Centre, we had acquired Marianne Green—who became dedicated to the cause as she helped to type much of the correspondence. Kay Keller, who is a meticulous bookkeeper became equally involved. In addition to being the national secretary and secretary of what was now the Victoria branch of the society, Leigh continued to collaborate in the production of the newsletter; travelling from the Island when necessary. Deborah remained the executive secretary and my administrative assistant. If the society had been obliged to hire someone to write the many programs which Shaun did for us, we would have been bankrupt.

As another year went by, awareness mounted; we presented briefs to both the Federal and Provincial Governments. In due course we were fortunate in being able to welcome Dr. J.A.L. Gilbert of the Department of Medicine at the University of Alberta in Edmonton to our Advisory Board; and, soon after this, to our great satisfaction, a Hematologist from Quebec: Doctor Marion Salusinky-Sternbach, Deputy Medical Director of the Red Cross Blood Transfusion Service in Montreal.

From the very beginning it had been a great comfort to have Maureen Worobey as our representative in Northern B.C. Now we hoped to find willing, enthusiastic people in other provinces. Before long, an article in the Calgary Herald resulted in a letter from Mervyn and Dorothy Minish of Swan River, Manitoba. Since then, together with their daughter, Trish, who lives in Winnipeg, they have conscientiously represented the C.H.S.in that part of the country. Another daughter, Elizabeth, is invaluable to the society in Vancouver.

In 1985, by a sort of spontaneous combustion, the C.H.S. began to take off by itself. Membership quadrupled in the first three months of the year. Working groups were established in a few centres; we had members in four countries. There were segments on Hemochromatosis on five Canadian television programs, as well as a poor but quite useful dramatization in one episode of ''Saint Elswhere''. Doctor Gerry Growe, a prominent Vancouver

Hematologist, was featured in a good interview with the Vancouver Sun, and Doctor Steinbrecher on BCTV. Both Doctor Hayden and Doctor Steinbrecher gave excellent account of themselves in radio interviews, and I participated in several programs with Tom as exhibit A on television. With the kind co-operation of the Surrey Memorial Hospital, Richie Nay was shown on CBC, undergoing a phlebotomy performed by Doctor Barrie Flather of Surrey.

There were times when we really, sincerely believed that, with every television program or radio interview we were nearer to licking the monster, IRON. . . . But we were never permitted to remain complacent for long. Every time someone died of HH, it was our personal loss—our personal failure. We could not be doing our jobs properly if there were still so many delayed or incorrect diagnoses. There were also the disheartening and frustrating cases of diagnosed patients who were unable to arrange for phlebotomies; the hardships of hospital user fees, which many who were too sick to work and who were required to pay for four or five venesections a month, found a tremedous drain. There remained the difficulty of persuading many a physician that HH was a serious business and that first-degree relatives should be tested.

Most disheartening of all was the tragedy of interrupted or discontinued therapy. Once bloodletting has commenced, iron stores reaccumulate at a faster rate than before, and—in order to avoid tissue damage—the removal of excess iron by venesection (or blood-letting) must take place at a rate calculated to remove the iron more quickly that reloading can occur. If it was distressing that many people were not being bled on a regular basis, it was horrifying to learn of some of the consequences of patients being told that they were cured or in "remission". In hereditary Hemochromatosis (HH), treatment is ongoing for life, although there comes a time when perhaps three or four phlebotomies a year will suffice. One woman was found to be in such poor health after a whole year without therapy that her doctor, trying to compensate for twelve months of neglect, bled her until she went into shock.

We could, however, do no more than were doing already. The society had become a twenty-four-hour-a-day, all-consuming undertaking. We could not afford an office and, as our home remained the headquarters of the society, Tom and I seldom ate a meal without interruption. Time changes from province to province in Canada, and the possibility of cheaper calls at certain times, meant that the telephone rang from before dawn until after eleven at night. It was not unusual to eat our evening meal as we listened; chewing and swallowing between sentences as we responded. And we would not have had it otherwise. As Dr. Steinbrecher said to me one day when I was feeling somewhat frazzled, "Well, isn't this what you wanted?"

I did. I had gone into this with my eyes open. I wanted to find EVERYONE who was at risk. Every diagnosis, every new member, every new entry in the registry, meant that I was getting closer to that goal; but I was becoming increasingly aware of my own inadequacy. I felt ashamed that I couldn't be all things to all people, at the same time.

As I sat at the dining room table, night after night, the food turned to sawdust in my mouth as I heard one tragic account after another. How familiar the stories were. I railed at the situation which existed; I writhed at the futility of it all! What an unworthy vessel I was. . . . !

Then something would happen to make me feel better. Was I not better than nothing at all? A letter from Mona Hogg of Delta, B.C. arrived on a day when I was feeling particularly worthless. She wrote:

"I would like to thank you most sincerely for information and counsel which, I have no doubt whatsoever, will prove to have saved the life of more than one person in my husband's family.

His diagnosis came only after seven years of miserable ill-health and even when he started treatment, no mention was made of the fact that the disease could be hereditary. We were told that it was rare and that very little was known about it. . . . We can only be thankful that an article in the Vancouver Sun, (sent to us by a friend) led us to the society, as subsequent tests proved that his brother and an uncle have Hemochromatosis and two nephews are at risk. We are writing to as many relatives as we can, and would appreciate it if you could let us have a few more brochures to pass on to them."

A letter from Denise Wiggins in Victoria could always make me feel better.

"I have read "Iron" with much interest and am part way

through it again. . . . . How foolish we are to accept symptoms as
'natural' when, if they persist, they are far from it!. . . . Thank
you for your never-ending search on our behalf.''

Some of the letters were tragic in the extreme. . . .

''Thank you for your very prompt response to my letters. After
seeing you on CTV during Christmas, 1985, and receiving your
brochure and 'Iron booklet' on this disorder, what you have done
for me has given me new hope and a certain peace of mind which
no words can possible describe. I am afraid my will or determination to live, or at least to find out what was happeneing to me,
was broken a few years ago and I've just been trying to hang on.
Things have been slipping from my grasp, past the point of
anger, past the point of despair, to the stage where my life had
become one of true apathy. . . . I believe I have suffered due to a
kindly family physician who was simply unaware or inadequate
to deal with my problem.

''I am changing doctors.

''. . . . I hope to write again and much better when or if I ever
feel well again.''

If all I could do was to provide a shoulder to cry on, I'd willingly offer that shoulder. I remembered all too vividly a time
when I felt like hurling myself into a moonlit swimming pool.
H.C. of New Westminster, British Columbia must have gone
through a great deal before writing.

Sometimes we would have guests to dinner and I would have
to excuse myself and go upstairs to talk on the 'phone there. Ex-
asperated after the third or fourth time I had been obliged to do
this, friends would try to reason with me. . . . ''You can't go on
like this, Marie. . . . Take the 'phone off the hook or turn on the
answering machine. . . . You shouldn't make yourself available at
meal times!''

But the truth of it was that, since I had returned to work, we ate
so late that people could be forgiven for expecting me to have fin-
ished by that time. I had gone back because certain very disquieting signs had long since made me accept the fact that the
''holiday'' was over. There were days when Tom's hands were
so bad that they locked on the steering wheel when he was driv-
ing; it became difficult for him to get his wallet out of a back

pocket. He tried to hide from me the fact that angina pain kept him awake at night. When he arrived home from work, his face was pinched and grey. To make matters worse, he had developed a rash on his face which, in addition to being an embarrasssment to him, was extremely painful at times.

I tried hard to be as loving and supportive as I could. Whenever possible, I tried to arrange a work schedule which made it possible for me to see him off in the mornings and be there for him when he came back. But, somehow my part-time work grew into full-time, and finally I was managing another store and working some twelve-hour days and seven day weeks. Back in Victoria, I had considered my work week long —but there had been Sundays and public holidays to look forward to. Imperceptibly, however, shopping malls on the mainland had been increasing shopping hours, and employees were no sooner resigned to working Sundays, when it was made known that the stores would open on public holidays, too, with very few exceptions.

I would have given anything to have been able to get off the treadmill but, as Tom's health declined, I was terrified of losing the security which the job offered me and, paradoxically, the fact that I was holding down a well-paid job, comforted Tom while it distressed him. He, too, read the writing on the wall. . . .

When he had returned to work so that I could stay at home, he had given me a wonderful gift. He had made it possible for me to do what I wanted so passionately to do—but at a dreadful cost to himself. Within three years his own health had deteriorated to an degree that is almost irreparable. Because of his knowledge, he had tackled the most intricate and exacting work. Because of his limitations, he was slower and had had to push himself harder to keep up with younger and fitter colleagues. As worsening arthritis further crippled his hands, the stress of holding his own increased; and as the joint disease in his feet imposed further restrictions, preventing the exercise which is so essential to the diabetic, the endless battle to control ever-rising bloodsugar levels became and still is a losing battle.

Nocturnal angina robbed him of sleep. I came home from work one day and noticed that the bed had been slept on; however as Tom had met me at the door with his usual smile of welcome and had made Shaun promise not to tell me that he had had to bring his father home from work in the middle of the afternoon, I was not concerned at the time. But is was not long before I was obliged to remember the incident. Tom spent part of December, 1985, in the Intensive Care Unit of Shaughnessy hospital, and a heart attack in December of 1986 landed him in ICU once more; this time in Richmond.

1986 had been not been an easy year. The society had expanded considerably by the summer, which had been an exhilarating season but a hard one. Expo had brought over twenty million visitors to British Columbia, no small percentage of them, it seemed, to visit with some of the volunteers upon whom I had learned to depend. Some of these ladies still tried loyally to give what time they could, to the urgent task of dealing with correspondence and other vital business; having to do that while coping with house guests and mentally fighting the greater attraction of the spectacular fair on our doorstep. But we soon had a greater backlog of work than Deb and I were able to deal with and some of our most ambitious projects did not come back on stream for some months.

Ever since I had returned to work, my dear friend, Marianne, had adhered to a strict routine. There just wasn't time any more for me to sit at the word-processor, writing letters. Instead, I would scribble my way through as many replies as possible and Marianne, who could decipher in the most miraculous way what I had written, would call at the store to collect the work, go home and type it, and then bring it back to me—more often than not on the same day. An excellent arrangement, until Marianne had to go for eye surgery.

I had for some time been corresponding with Roberta Crawford of Palm Beach, Florida, founder and President of the Iron Overload Diseases Association Inc. Despite the fact that she suffered from Hemochromatosis, herself, she seemed to be doing a magnificent job. Her publication, "Ironic Blood," was professional and informative. It was a source of great inspiration—as was "Hemochromatosis Awareness," Margit Krikker's newsletter. How difficult it was to give my own members everything I wanted to.

Sometimes it was all like a nightmare. I couldn't cope but I dared not quit. Things had had reached the stage when I felt guilty if I took a break from Hemochromatosis. When I could not afford to send a newsletter or was prevented by other circumstances from writing one, I spent so much time worrying about it that I soon realized that it was easier to get on with the job and get it behind me. Once, when I was just too sick to carry on, Shaun was obliged to write to every member, apologizing on my behalf for my silence.

There were times when I confronted my obsession sanely and sensibly and admitted to myself that I would have to slow down. Tom Rogerson advised me not to try so hard. "Just sit back and let things grow by themselves," he said. And for a while I did try. But it would take only one letter from someone who suffered **needlessly**, to set me off again. What got to me again and again was the fact that what had happened to Tom and countless others had been **preventable**!

The cruel irony of the whole darned iron thing was enough to drive me crazy. I combed supermarket shelves for products which did not contain added iron and searched for bread without sugar. Some products are not only already enriched; they contain additional iron. Why should every wheat product be fortified with iron?

I wrote to the Federal Minister of Health, Monique Begin, complaining that hemochromatotics were hastening their own death by eating breakfast cereal and was considerably upset by her reply that they could eat granola. To my mind, that suggestion smacked of Marie Antoinette's famed reponse regarding the eating of cake because there was no bread. Did Madame Begin not realize, I wondered, that granola was loaded with sugar or honey and many of these people were diabetic?

When a cardiologist at Shaugnessy hospital in Vancouver gave me a list of foods high in iron, drawing my attention to the fact that there was more iron in certain baby formulae than in any other item on the list, he did not realize that, in giving me something else to fret about, he was hastening my early demise. I tortured myself wondering. . . . what effect would such a diet have on an infant who was homozygous for Hemochromatosis? A woman telephoned my one morning at work to tell me excitedly that she had found iron reduced cookies which she was about to take home to her husband who suffered cruelly from cirrhosis of the liver, induced by iron. Now I had a new worry. What was to be done about the wording on food labels? She had in fact bought cookies containing "reduced iron"—a form more readily assimilated into the body! How could we ever win when so much conspired against us?

I experienced periods of intense despair which could only be alleviated by action, and at such times I would bombard the media.

A milestone was reached when Macleans were finally prevailed upon to feature an article in October, 1986, because, not long after that, the Medical Post—part of the same group—devoted one-and-a-half pages with full-colour photographs to HH. As a result of this, Doctor Valberg received numerous letters from Canadian physicians, which was excellent as far as educating the doctor was concerned. Unfortunately, however, the address of the society was not given in either of the articles and it was only due to tenacity and determination that some people did manage to contact us.

Among those who did, were two gentlemen who would prove very valuable to us. The first, Bill Millholland of Sarnia, Ontario, is now a representative of the CHS in that area. The story of the second, Eugene Boyko of Richmond, B.C., is an interesting one. Upon reading the Maclean's article, he knew at last what had been wrong with him for many years and, having virtually diagnosed himself, lost no time in getting his physician to carry out the necessary tests. His suspicions proved to be correct and now, as he puts it, he is grateful and wants to "give something back." He was recently elected National Vice-President of the Canadian Hemochromatosis Society.

With apologies to Dickens and the "Tale of Two Cities", it was the worst of times; but in many ways it was the best of times. Kay Keller, who had added the task of "book sales co-ordinator" to her other responsibilities, found it awe-inspiring but highly amusing that, whenever I was at my wits end, I would pray about it, and the problem would resolve itself.

One night, as I was wrestling with the seemingly impossible

task of having to write a letter in French to someone in Montreal, I said almost desperately: " I don't wish anyone to be afflicted because of me, but I do wish the Lord would send me a Frenchman with Hemochromatosis!" And the next morning, there he was at my door. . . . a dapper little man from Quebec, a new member for the society, well-educated and willing; capable even of translating words like "chondrocalcinosis"!

Among the answers to my prayers was Frances Olsen, who volunteered to bring our cardex up-to-date, and Richie Nay, who would help with things like manning an exhibit or selling books. And should we not be grateful that now it was not unusual to hear of two, new diagnoses in one week!

Perhaps we were getting there, after all. . . .

But my prayers for Tom were **not** being answered. The time had long since passed when he could even walk through a shopping mall.

On the first Sunday in December I did not have to work. Tom and Shaun were absorbed in a project of mutual interest, Deborah was out shopping and I—as had become my custom when I needed a quiet place to work—sat outside of Shaun's house, in the Hammy, addressing Christmas cards. Those cards were never mailed. . . . and last Christmas I didn't send any either. . . .

Deb had just returned when I realised that I needed an address which only she could give me. I walked into their livingroom in time to see Shaun bend over his father in great concern. . . .

Prayers are not always answered in the way we want them to be. The events of the next few weeks would hardly seem what I had asked for. Nevertheless, in time I could only thank God for a miraculous set of circumstances without which Tom could not have made it. If we had been at our own home at the time, I could not have got him down three sets of stairs and into our car. . . . if Deb's car had not been in the open garage, not fifty feet from where Tom was slumped in the chair. . . . if Shaun had not been home to take Tom. . . . and if we had not been visiting the children, a mere stone's throw from the hospital. . . . !

CHAPTER FIVE

WHEN TOM AND I MOVE, THE SOCIETY MOVES WITH US. Like a snail with its house on its back, we take the CHS wherever we go. And, with files under our bed and the computer in one corner of the bedroom, we lived with the children for three months after Tom's heart attack.

All that time I wrestled with the consuming anger which threatened to drive even gratitude from my heart.

A despairing, agonizing fury robbed me of sleep and left me pounding my pillow with clenched fists as I deliberately tortured myself by reliving all that Tom (and I) had already suffered because of IRON. I would watch him in the hospital as he patiently waited to pass the next hurdle and the next; take his first shower; walk around the ward. He came home and longed for the day when he could go outside. Every day wonderful people from the home care service came to take his pulse, only to go away shaking their heads because it was so slow.

When he was finally allowed to go for his first walk out of doors, it was an agony for him because of the crippling arthritis in his feet. Reading was little pleasure to him as he could barely hold a book; his hands hurt so much. No matter how rigidly we stuck to the prescibed diet, his blood sugar soared. . . . and, as it did, so did my anger. . . .

It was probably because of the need to channel my own frustration into positive action that I made up my mind, almost grimly, that if Tom lived to see another birthday, the whole country would be told of the ravages of iron overload. There were about 75,000 Canadians who could die if they were not found; thousands might suffer **unnecessarily** as a result of abysmal ignorance, but not if I could help it. May 25, 1987 would be Hemochromatosis Awareness Day in Canada because of what Tom had suffered, and, if one life was saved, someone, somewhere would have cause to be thankful for that day.

I knew that it was going to be done but I needed just that extra little shove to get me over the brow of the hill. For a while I could only scheme and ponder; nervously trying just my toe in the water; not quite ready to dive, in case it was too cold. Then, one evening, just before supper, Deb called me upstairs to take a call on her 'phone. I spoke into the receiver and a young girl's voice responded. Her name was Nancy, she said. In a well-controlled voice which, by its very calmness, betrayed the underlying emotion, she told me that her father had just died of Hemochromatosis and her family had requested that donations in lieu of flowers be sent to the CHS. She was just checking for the correct mailing address.

Somehow I managed to speak with equal matter-of-factness as I gave her the information she wanted, and succeeded reasonably well until she said something about his only recently having been diagnosed, "just five years too late!"

I groaned as we talked further and cried myself to sleep that night. The family lived in North Vancouver. How was it possible? We had been active on the Lower Mainland of British Columbia for several years and yet we had never reached this man. Her mother's name was Charmian, she had said. He father's was Jack. I felt that I knew them personally. I shared the sadness in that home and suffered the most terrible sense of hopelesssness. As I had done so many times before, I reproached myself for not having done my job properly. . . . I had been given the shove I needed. . . . !

It turned out to be not only one day of awareness but a whole week. Mayor Gil Blair of Richmond, British Columbia, was the first to sign a proclamation and it was at the suggestion of his office that the week of May 25 to 31 was designated. Had Mayor

Blair and the corporation of Richmond not been amenable, we should probably have abandoned the whole undertaking. The fact that they did so, is due to an incredible set of circumstances.

When I told Tom Mark of CJOR radio in Vancouver about my plans for an awareness day, he proved to be a sympathic listener and was quite obviously intrigued by the fact that anyone could actually be adversely affected by too much iron. He taped an interview with me, in which I explained what Hemochromatosis was, told of the tragic consequences of iron overload and emphasized the need for awareness in order to achieve diagnosis before it was too late. The interview was broadcast very early on the following Sunday morning, to be followed by the expected number of phone calls. Then, having complied with the initial requests for information, were were mystified when, some days later, there was a further spate of inquiries. We could not account for the sudden renewal of interest, as we did not know that the interview had been broadcast a second time.

On the day on which Tom, Kay Keller and I went down to the mayor's office in Richmond for the signing of the proclamation, Mayor Blair confessed: "You know, at first I wasn't going to do this. . . . We get so many of these requests and I'd never heard of this. . . . this. . . . Hemochromatosis. . . . But then, last Sunday, I was still in bed and I heard some woman talking about it on the radio and that convinced me!"

I still haven't been able to confess that I was the woman. I can only be grateful for the co-incidence; for the fact that the tape was played a second time. Once Richmond had given the stamp of approval, other corporations followed suit and, in due course proclamations were signed by the mayors of almost every city in Canada; even by the Government of British Columbia.

There were times when I could not believe that I could have let myself and my friends in for such a far-fetched, seemingly hair-brained scheme. Strangely, however, no-one seemed terribly taken aback and no-one tried to talk me out of it. Kay Keller, sympathetic of the fact that we were house-bound, had taken over the banking for the society and had become a regular visitor since Tom's heart attack. When she arrived one day to find me puzzling over the most efficient way in which to personalize the hundreds of letters which would have to be sent to mayors, she picked up one I had already written, studied it for a minute and then said: "I'll do it!"

She did, too. I would spend a few hours every morning at the library, scribbling down the names and addresses of more mayors and the afternoon Kay would fetch them. By next day, each new batch was ready for mailing.

The first nine we found, all worked in or in close association with the offices of mayors to whom we had written. Not one of those people would have known that HH was hereditary and none would have had themselves checked had it not been for our writing. One woman, whose brother-in-law had died of Hemochromatosis had considered the similarity of her husband's symptoms "pure co-incidence"! Nine people meant nine **families** to be monitored.

The unexpected success we achieved in the Maple Ridge area of British Columbia must, however, be attributed to more than co-incidence. In every letter Kay and I made mention of our "enclosed green brochure" which, we said, would provide further information. Somehow, one letter was mailed without that enclosure, and it just happened to be the one to Maple Ridge. Some days later I received a telephone call from Alderman Roman Evancic, who informed me that the council meeting at which the requested awareness day proclamation was to be read, was to be televised that evening. He would like to have a few more details before the time.

It was he who remarked that the omission of the brochure had perhaps been providential. We talked a long time because of this and, that evening, as the telecast went out to viewers in that region, there was quite a dramatic turn of events. Referring to the proclamation, Alderman Evancic supported it by telling of how Hemochromatosis had affected someone in his own family.

Before long I was obliged to appeal for help in a newsletter and was overwhelmed by the response. As was to be expected, among the first to respond were Betty Campbell in Guelph and the Minishes in Manitoba; their daughter, Elizabeth, was already involved in British Columbia. Then came a 'phone call from Kay and Norm Belanger who did such a fantastic job, covering from Port Mellon in the South to Powell River in the North, that within seven months a full-fledged branch of the society had been established on the Sunshine Coast.

What we had not anticipated was the number of people, many with absolutely no genetic reason for doing so, who volunteered to promote awareness because they believed that it was imperative to do so. Newsletters are sent to hospitals across the country and some of the most valuable assistance came from hospital personnel. For instance, in Rocky Mountain House, Alberta, Ileene Hulberg—director—and her fellow health record technicians, arranged for Mayor Lou Soppit to sign the proclamation at the hospital, from which the program of awareness for the area was launched.

Eugene Boyko, his diagnosis confirmed by a liver biopsy, and by now having had his first few phlebotomies, acted as coordinator and made our posters. His wife, Del, took charge of assigning to volunteers the sort of jobs for which they were most suited.

As the big day approached, parcels consisting of posters and information leaflets had to be sent to every municipalty in which the awareness week was to be observed. Deb provided a beautifully typed , personalized letter of thanks to accompany each parcel. Marie Crellin and other friends and neighbours helped Tom to stuff envelopes. When the time came, they sat in shopping malls handing out leaflets or called on medical laboratories, emergency departments of hospitals and doctors' offices, distributing literature and putting up posters.

We compiled an album to preserve the many proclamations which we could not afford to have framed. One is missing. It was arranged with the Mayor's office in London, Ontario, that the proclamation signed in that city, be presented to Doctor Leslie Valberg, Dean of Medicine at the University of Western Ontario, as our tribute for his magnificent dedication to Hemochromatosis research.

I had a special reason for wanting to do a particularly good job on the North Shore in Vancouver; but, somehow, that was one area in which we were obviously going to have a problem. Until one day, my young friend Nancy called. "I'd like to cover the North Shore area," she said. "Because of my father, I want people to know about this. . . . !"

Help appeared from another unexpected quarter. I was playing the organ in the Bay in downtown Vancouver, when I heard a voice behind me say: "I thought I recognized you!" There stood Debbie Norton, my very first volunteer from Victoria, whom I had not seen for many years. She had recently moved to the mainland and immediately offered her help in the West End.

A friend, whose father-in-law had played in Tom's band more than fifteen years before, made herself available in Oakdale and Hamilton. . . . A grandmother of a hemochromatotic family would work in another part of Ontario. . . . and so it went. . . .

I never once asked for money but donations came when they were most needed.

* * * *

Some incredible stories came out of the awareness week. I had already witnessed so much suffering and had heard of such tragedy that I thought I knew it all. How wrong I was. . . .

Among the most disturbing were the accounts of the unbelievable, culpable nonsense some people had been led by their family physicians to accept as fact. One of most astounding, as far as I am concerned, was the explanation that one woman's deceased brother had contracted Hemochromatosis in a Japanese prisoner of war camp. "Our doctor," she informed me, "says that many Canadians had this done to them by the Japanese!" Because of this erroneous belief, parallel signs in other family members would not be investigated.

For nine years I had been assimilating knowledge on a steady, ongoing basis. Suddenly, as a result of the intense concentration on HH and the sudden bombardment of information, I was learning more in the last year than in all the other years put together. I discovered, among other things, a great deal about myself and my approach.

For example, when I wrote "Iron. . . . the other side of the story!", I attempted to point out the danger of delayed diagnosis and listed such complications as I deemed necessary to enable the average reader to seek medical advice. However, when I sent a pre-print of the booklet to Dr. Valberg for his criticism, I confessed that I had tried to focus on the optimistic. There were some aspects of iron overload which I found so dreadful that I could make no reference to them.

"I didn't want to make it too scary," I admitted, and now I wonder whether I misconstrued his reply. . . . "You don't have to make it scary. . . it's scary enough!"

In the October 27, 1986 edition of Maclean's, a week after the publication of the article on Hemochromatosis, a Toronto woman whose friend had succumbed to HH the previous year, wrote in a letter to the editor that the article had been informative but had not adequately described the "intense suffering experienced by victims of this terrible disease". In another paragraph she referred to it as a "truly dreadful disease".

I agreed wholeheartedly but still could never bring myself to tell it as it was, for fear of terrifying anyone who was already afflicted; always hoping against hope that every person I dealt with would be among the fortunate—the ones who were diagnosed before his or her condition was hopeless. Perhaps if I had painted the true Dorian Gray, the media might have been provoked earlier into helping me.

One involvement I had steered clear of was that of esophageal varices or enlarged veins in the throat. To me this was just too horrible to contemplate. I now consider that I erred in this omission from my booklet for I now believe that to shrink from all mention of this complication was sheer cowardice. It was simply another manifestation of my early employment of euphemism. Tom's mother would not have flinched.

Since the time when one of my earliest correspondents had decribed to me her husband's death as the result of a massive hemorrhage, I had added to my files, several accounts which were similar. If I had written about them, I might have done much good.

This became painfully clear to me when an elegantly dressed woman came by the table at which Tom and I were sitting in the Oakridge Shopping Centre on the third day of the awareness week. She stopped to talk for a while and surprised us by actually knowing about HH. Moreover,having been made aware of the disorder by the death of her husband's father she had bought my booklet at Eaton's in Richmond. Happily, she informed us, no-one else in the family was afflicted or even at risk. They were all fine except her husband who was very ill; he had unfortunately just been hospitalized because of enlarged veins in the throat; due,it was suspected, to medication which had been administered to him some years previously. Neither she nor her husband had ever thought to mention to the doctor in charge of her husband's case that there was a family history of HH.

I restrained myself with difficulty from offering any comment other than to entreat her to have her sons checked. If their grandfather had been afflicted, I pointed out, the boys' father would have to be a carrier. I could only suggest that she tell the doctor about her father-in-law without delay.

Shortly after this encounter in the shopping mall, I met face-to-face for the first time, two people who had seldom been out of my thoughts since that telephone call several months before. Nancy had brought her mother to see us. I took an instant liking to them both and resolved to keep in touch. Recently Charmian, convinced that others might profit from her story, gave me permission to print it. Why I regard it as one of the most tragic of all the experiences which have been shared with me, is obvious. Why I have repeated, over and over again "if only there had been awareness long ago!" will also become very clear.

This is her story as she wrote it. I am grateful to her for allowing me to include it in this book.

Jack and I married in 1949 in Regina, Sask. after knowing one another since Grade 6. I guess what attracted me at the time was how much older and wiser he seemed than all the other boys of his age. Of course now I know that he didn't have the energy to keep up with them so he spent long hours reading and was very knowledgeable about world affairs etc. etc. Jack joined Sea Cadets in his early teens and had to pass a medical but the Doctor was a family friend and an Urologist who didn't look too deeply for anything wrong.

In 1945, Jack joined the Wartime Navy and again had to pass a medical but they were put through like cattle in a huge hall and the doctor did put him aside but in the end let him pass. His pulse rate at this point was 52 and has always been slow. In 1951 he rejoined the Navy and on the strength of all his other medicals he was admitted. At this time we were in Halifax and left there in 1960 for Victoria. It was there that Jack had a fainting spell and was thoroughly examined by many doctors who discovered that he had a congenital heart block which meant the communication between brain and heart was not complete and his heart beat as an involuntary muscle with no impulses getting through from the brain. So with this diagnosis I felt it explained his lack of energy and enthusiasm for anything other than his work. In 1965 we were back in Halifax and Jack was Executive Officer of a ship at sea.

He had just returned from a voyage when he complained of chest pain and was admitted to the Naval Hospital. The next day he suffered a cerebral embolism with left hemiparesis and it was touch and go for many days whether he would live. However he recovered and went back to work full time after 3 or 4 months of parttime. In 1967 he had another cerebral episode and this time was flown to the Service Hospital in Ottawa. There thoroughly tested and returned saying that he was to go back on his anticoagulants for life. They had tried to stop them because while he was on them his medical category was "D"—meaning he was frozen at this present promotion level and could never advance in rank. However he decided to stay in the Navy until his required retirement time and we had a lovely 2 years in Hawaii from 1969 to 1971 and then spent the last 2 years of his service time in Victoria.

In 1973 he tried for and got a job in Vancouver with the Coast Guard and became the Officer in Charge of Vancouver Vessel Traffic Control Centre which he retained until his second retirement last October. His health, of course, deteriorating all the time. In 1976 marked cerebral atrophy was noted and in 1980, he suffered Thrombophlebitis in his leg and had heart fibrillations, going on to having a pacemaker inserted. By this time he had gout, high tone hearing loss, marked hand tremor and prostatism.

The summer of 1982 was a nightmare with terrible mood swings and irrational behavior, the end result being a diagnosis of Diabetes, to be controlled by twice daily insulin injections, 4 time daily Glucometer readings and the addition of Lithium to control the mood swings. An enlarged liver was also noted at this time. He stabilized out for the next few years but had no energy and managed his job because of strong support from all his staff at work and me at home. I had always felt that if I hadn't been a nurse and caught all his symptoms before they became too bad he would have died much earlier from any one of his conditions.

We went on a motor trip last June to Saskatchewan and it was a nightmare for me. He seemed completely oblivious to his weird behaviour and lack of mental stability. He went into insulin shock the first night back, recovered and returned to his job for about 6 weeks and then was unable to continue after mid August.

At the beginning of August Dr. Lang began to suspect Hemochromatosis because of the color his skin. He had the blood tests done and they were wildly positive. Iron—203, TIBC—231, % Sat. 88, Ferritin 660.8. However the final diagnosis could not be made until after a liver biopsy which needed a specialist and he was on holidays. After it was finally done in day care at the hospital, it was of course positive. So the phlebotomies were started weekly (15 in all with one being done the day of his death) and his energy level took another plunge.

It was all he could do to get out of bed in the morning, dress himself and just sit in a chair all day. His appetite was gone and his concentration was zero. He couldn't even read. He would be watching games on TV but he didn't know the score. There was marked edema in his ankles and feet and around his waist making walking very difficult. On December 10th, I had been shopping and came home to find him in bed complaining of a stomach ache. He was admitted to hospital and they decided it was the edema and started him on large doses of diuretics. It was pitiful. He never made it to the bathroom, all dignity was gone. He stopped eating even when fed. I didn't see how he could keep going. I phoned my sons, one in Germany the other in Halifax and told them the end was near. He had a wonderfully bright 3 days (the last of the adrenalin being released) before he vomited blood the night of January 2nd and 4 hours later he was gone. The autopsy showed that he had a massive upper gastrointestinal hemorrhage secondary to esophageal varices. He had 1) Hemochromatosis with cirrhosis, pancreatic atrophy, cardiomegaly, testicular atrophy and ascites. 2) Aortic valve damage. 3) Myocardial degeneration in left ventricle. 4) Old renal infarcts. 5) Old right cerebral infarct. 6) Old and recent splenic infarcts.

He was born July 29, 1926 and died January 2, 1987.

* * * *

Several physicians participated in the awareness program. Dr. Steinbrecher presented a talk on HH on CJOR in Vancouver, which did an enormous amount for us, and Doctors Michael Raine and Macolm Brigden very kindly joined me on the Joe Easingwood Show in Victoria. One Vancouver woman told me that, fearing that the reception might not be good on the mainland, she had travelled all the way to Vancouver Island to be able hear them. In Gibson's Landing, Kay Belanger acted as the interviewer on local cablevision, while Dr.J.F. Hourigan and I had Tom and Kay's husband, Norm, on hand to back up our statements with personal experience.

To "kick off" the awareness week, Dr. Michael Hayden and I were guests on a CKNW phone-in, talk show in Vancouver. I found one of the calls particlarly interesting although I knew that it was going to cause me some stress. It was from a woman whose father had just been diagnosed at the age of 87.

There was little that could be done for him, it seeemed, but some good would still come of his diagnosis. Because of this, his family would be forewarned. The provocative part of it was that the man had been a blood donor until the age of 65, after which he was no longer permitted to donate blood.

Dr. Hayden explained that it was probably because of the fact that the iron had been eliminated from his system for many years that Hemochromatosis had manifested itself so late in his life. Many nights after that, when I could not sleep, I wrestled with the problem of whether it might not be advisable to check potential blood donors early, before their first donation, in order to establish whether they were at risk. If one knew of the potential for accumulating iron when bloodgiving ceased, surely one could then go for a phlebotomy at intervals, to prevent the complications of Hemochromatosis.

* * * *

I don't think anyone knew why, at the stage when there was going to be only one day of awareness, I had particularly chosen May 25. Tom sat outside, listening to us over the car radio and, as I pictured him out there, the even greater significance of this day washed over me.

It was twelve years since Tom had been given twelve weeks. . . . !

I was so grateful and suddenly so concerned about his brother. Surely awareness, like charity, began at home. Certain things I had noticed about Selby at our last meeting, two years before, had disquieted me to the extent that I had mentioned them to Tom. Selby had been in one hospital for some time but, right at that at that moment was seriously ill in another, to which he had been taken with pneumonia. At that moment he was in the very hospital in which Tom had been diagnosed and first treated.

I could stand it no longer.

Taking extreme care to word my letter in a way which would not offend, I wrote to Selby's family doctor. I told him how Hemochromatosis had devastated Tom and said that I had I had detected in his brother significant signs with which I had become familiar in nine years of meeting with other afflicted people. I then explained about the week of awareness in Canada, and apologizing for what might appear to be interference, explained that this was what had prompted me to write. Selby had suffered for years from bleeding hemorrhoids which might have affected the results of tests done previously. Recent surgery had, however, corrected that problem, perhaps with the result that iron loading was now excessive. Would he not please oblige us by carrying out the tests once more? In conclusion, I mentioned that the eminent authority on iron overload, Professor Bothwell, who had been instrumental in saving Tom's life, just happened to be connected with the hospital in which my brother-in-law was recuperating from pneumonia. I felt sure that the professor would be only too happy to be consulted if there was any problem.

Selby is fortunate in having a doctor who keeps an open mind. As we kept score of new diagnoses which resulted from our awareness week, he, Selby, was number seventy-four!

CHAPTER SIX

THE REPERCUSSIONS OF LAST MAY ARE STILL BEING FELT and will continue to be felt for as long as the Canadian Hemochromatosis Society exists.

The immediate results have already necessitated the restructuring of our whole mode of operation. We have expanded into parts of this country—and others—in which we were unknown before; we have members and people willing to represent us in areas where we formerly had a very low profile; we seem now to enjoy an enhanced credibility where goverment and the medical profession are concerned; we have the knowledge that, across this country and some other parts of the world, there are people who may live longer and enjoy a better quality of life because of our efforts; the influence of the CHS is certainly more widespread than we could have believed one year ago.

We have come a long way since the days when our efforts were mainly directed towards finding enough people to hold a meeting; we have progressed considerably since our chief objectives were simply to correct the many misconceptions surrounding HH. The Canadian Hemochromatosis Society has six branches across Canada, members in nine countries and affiliates in four of them. The newest of the branches are headed up by Maureen Worobey,(B.C. NORTH), Pat and David Fleming,(B.C. INTERIOR); an ONTARIO branch has recently been formed by Sally and George Hutson.

Hemochromatosis is certainly now a word better known to the

media. An interview I had with Mike Bernard of the Canadian Press Association wire service was picked up by newspapers across the country, with very few exceptions, and resulted in my being contacted by a radio network which has its headquarters in California. And as the first nine people who were positively affected by our campaign were all employees in Mayors' offices, perhaps some municipal health authorities are now also aware of HH. Large corporations, for example B.C. Ferries, and B.C. Tel made literature available to members of staff, as did some branches of the Bay and Woodwards. The Richmond Savings Credit Union not only distributed our pamphlet to all clients and members of staff; they did their own photocopying and saved us a considerable expense.

Perhaps the awareness will be ongoing. . . . !

But we have still only scratched the surface!

As a result of the awareness week in 1988, we have achieved, to date, 523 new diagnoses. . . But what is 523 against the desired 75,000? We try to comfort ourselves with the thought that an additional 523 individuals may live because of our efforts. And when we think of cases known to us where there are three, four, and as many as nine diagnosed members in one family, we hope that we may perhaps have had an impact on many of whom we are as yet unaware. At the time of going to press, the Government of British Columbia has signed a proclamation for the 1988 week of awareness and it is expected that some of the other provincial governments will follow suit.

523 new diagnoses!. . . It has a good ring to it! But now we have a new problem. Many patients who have been undergoing treatment for a number of years are finding that their doctors are growing tired and somewhat dismayed at the prospect of a seemingly endless program of treatment—and who can blame them..? Because many physicians do not want new HH patients, not all of the newly-diagnosed are able to make satisfactory arrangements for phlebotomy therapy on an ongoing basis.

It is my sincere belief that Hemochromatosis may prove to be the scourge of the 21st century unless something is done now, by responsible governments, to combat it. In saying this I am not merely expressing my own opinion —there are physicians who are saying the same thing. The estimated prevalence has already reached alarming proportions. It is described in 'Ironic Blood' as "the secret, silent epidemic" which many countries are now taking very seriously. New York Senator D'Amato and Californian Representative Vic Fazio introduced joint resolutions in Congress last year, to ask President Reagan to proclaim an Awareness Day in the U.S.A. where, it is estimated, between 600,000 and 1,600,000 individuals are affected. 24-32 million Americans are carriers of the recessive gene.

In Canada, as in every other country to which these facts apply, first degree relatives of known probands have to be screened for their protection—and this won't happen until every medical practitioner recognizes the vital importance of this. Something will have to be done about the misleading wording on iron-fortified foods; the whole practice of enriching food with iron will have to be reviewed; iron supplements will have to carry a warning label and some sort of, efficient, large-scale screening program will have to be instituted to effect earlier diagnosis. Ideally spouses of known heterozygotes and homozygotes will be checked in order that offspring who inherit double genes for HH may be treated **before** they are affected.

Furthermore, there will have to be a more consistent program for the treatment of patients once they are diagnosed. . . . Some are bled in emergency departments of hospitals; others in doctors' rooms. In some places it is permissible for nurses to carry out venesections; in others it is mandatory to have a doctor in attendance. In Montreal the Red Cross does a splendid job of caring for the HH patient; in British Columbia the Red Cross is not licensed as a treatment centre. . . . just another example of how the system various across Canada.

523 new diagnoses. . . . ! That figure would undoubtedly have been higher if everyone who recognized the signs or who suddenly realized that HH in one family member meant that others were risk, had been fortunate enough to be given a test when it was requested.

If only everyone who WAS tested had been given the COR-RECT tests!

Nine years of my life have been invested in this. Nine years have been demanded of my children and their spouses, my grandchildren and anyone else who would be roped in. Almost as many years have been devoted by the wonderful people who have supported me in this crusade. We can do no more. . . .

* * * *

Up to the moment of writing, the Canadian Hemochromatosis Society receives no financial assistance from any source other than donations and since those who have suffered the ravages of HH will give anything to prevent similar suffering in loved ones, it is usually the same people who give, time and time again; believing, as we all do, that the only solution is to prevent, by timely diagnosis and treatment, the complications of what they, themselves, have inherited.

That they should have to do this, seems unfair; it is as though they are all required to pay twice.-- Firstly, in pain and suffering, in the loss of income as they become robbed of the capacity to work; in the tragic lack of the quality of life which could have been their due if excess iron had not taken from them so much of what makes the living worthwhile. Secondly, in assisting the society to carry on its work, they contribute financially to what should not have to be the responsibility of any patient. . . . namely, the education and enlightenment of so many members of the medical profession. . . .

EPILOGUE

FOR YEARS TOM HAD SUFFERED FROM ARRHYTHMIA. NOT long after his heart attack, he began to experience periods of such severe tachycardia (rapid heartbeat) that the chair on which he was sitting would vibrate. If he was lying down, the whole bed would shake. It became almost routine to rush him to emergency at Richmond General Hospital.

Depite this, and in defiance of his doctor's warning that his own failing health made the undertaking too hazardous, Tom,— greatly concerned about his ailing brother— insisted, in August, 1988 on travelling to South Africa. On our arrival, before we had cleared customs, he collapsed, and was taken to hospital by ambulance. We had been told two years previously in Vancouver that surgery was not possible; however, a quadruple by-pass was performed by Professor Robin Kinsley at the Morningside Clinic. By the Grace of God, despite the many other ravages of Hemochromatosis, his condition is no longer life-threatening.

It is quite wonderful to be able to go for a walk with him once more—when the joint disease in his feet, ankles, hips and knees permit this. . . . !

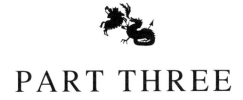

PART THREE

IRON—The Other Side of the Story

IRON

THE OTHER SIDE OF THE STORY!

DIABETES... ARTHRITIS... A TAN WHICH

NEVER FADES... CHRONIC FATIGUE...

ABDOMINAL PAIN... IMPOTENCE...

DIMINISHED LIBIDO... PREMATURE

MENOPAUSE... ARRHYTHMIA... CIRRHOSIS

OF THE LIVER...

can be the result of

TOO MUCH IRON!

DIABETES... ARTHRITIS... A TAN WHICH NEVER FADES...

CHRONIC FATIGUE... ABDOMINAL PAIN... IMPOTENCE...

could be signs of

HEMOCHROMATOSIS

The Insidious Killer

First printing: August, 1984
Updated March, 1988

CHAPTER ONE

HEMOCHROMATOSIS—The Insidious Killer

IT IS HORRIFYING TO CONTEMPLATE THAT IN EVERY AVER-age class of thirty, in every average school in this country, there could be three to five young people who are carriers of a crippling and potentially fatal genetic disorder—Hemochromatosis—and do not know it.

This hypothesis springs from an intensive nine-year study, a self-imposed project of my own, which has involved reading anything and everything pertaining to the subject, on which I could lay my hands; and personal interviews or correspondence with leading authorities as well as with many, many afflicted families. I am indebted to them all; but most particularly to those who have been willing to share experiences with me and who have so readily given me permission to use what they have told me.

In the face of what I have learned, I find only one thing more frustrating than having someone take an impressive tome from the bookshelf to point triumphantly to where it says something about an estimated incidence of 1 in 20,000 people— and that is to discover that the medical dictionary or book of reference makes no mention of Hemochromatosis at all! Some text books currently on sale and recommended for use by medical students are hopelessly out of date and too many physicians, having been led to believe that it is so rare, are not on the alert for signs of the disease. . . . because they simply do not expect to find them.

Recent genetic studies, based on families with the disease, indicate that hereditary Hemochromatosis is **the** most common, of genetic disorders while, paradoxically, the one that is most often dismissed as "rare". Because it so often goes unrecognised, it is rarely diagnosed before it is clinically manifest. Most of the suffering associated with the disease is preventable if potential victims are detected in time; and even when it has become symptomatic, many serious complications are reversible— but only by timely diagnosis and treatment.

Primary or hereditary Hemochromatosis (HH), also referred to as Idiopathic Hemochromatosis (IHC), is transmitted as an autosomal recessive disorder[i] and it is estimated that 10-13% of the Caucasian population are heterozygotes, or carriers.[ii] **Heterozygotes**, as **carriers**, do not, themselves, have the disease. **Homozygote** is the term used to describe those individuals who have HH because they have inherited **two** Hemochromatosis genes, one from each of their carrier parents.

Every child of a homozygote will be a carrier.

In 1977, the prevalence of homozygosity, estimated by Edwards et al, and in 1979 by Cartwright et al, was about one in three-hundred to one in five-hundred; an estimate supported by the finding of homozygosity in 1 in 333 Utahns (Cartwright et al), 1 in 400 Bretons (Beaumont et al, 1979), and, in an autopsy study, 1 in 500 Scots. (Mac Sween and Scott, 1973.) The estimates have risen considerably since then.

In some countries, for example AUSTRALIA, 16% of the population, or **one in every six or seven people is a carrier,** according to Bassett et al.

Originally, a considerable part of my own correspondence was with Canadians of Scottish origin, particularly in Alberta. During the last two years, however, I have been provided with the case histories of men, women and children of every European race. The Canadian Hemochromatosis Society has lately added a large number of Ukranians and even one Chinese man to its membership list; it is however not yet known whether his iron-overload was induced or of genetic origin. The hereditary form of the disease has long been regarded as affecting primarily Caucasians; consequently, available statistics are based on Caucasian studies. Research among non- Caucasians will possibly disprove yet another misconception.

Results of a study published in 1983 in the Canadian journal, Clinical and Investigative Medicine (Vol.6, no 3, pp 171-179) by S.T. Borwein, C.N. Ghent, P.R. Flanagan, M.J. Chamberlain and L.S. Valberg, under the title "Genetic and Phenotypic Expression of Hemochromatosis in Canadians"[iii] revealed that 11% of the Caucasian population of Canada are estimated to be carriers and that the disease frequency for homozygotes is estimated to be 1 in 333.

It is now generally accepted that **75,000 Canadians may die of Hemochromatosis if they are not found in time.** However, A new survey would probably show the existing estimate for Canada to be already outdated, as every paper presented by reseachers of other developed countries brings proof of rising numbers. When results of more recent studies were presented to the American College of Physicians in Washington, Corwin Q. Edwards, M.D., Associate Professor of Medicine at the University of Utah, reported a homozygote (two genes necessary to develop the full-blown disease) frequency of one in two hundred. Similarly, all other estimates were higher than those previously on record.

The figure for FRANCE, according to Beaumont et al, were similar to those for homozygotes in Canada, with one in ten estimated to be a carrier. Ollsson et al of SWEDEN, estimate that one person in every seven or eight carries one gene; one in two hundred Swedes has the genetic makeup to develop the deadly disease.

The findings of a group of SOUTH AFRICANS, published in the British Journal of Medical Genetics last year[xiv], is of significance in every country with population groups of the same genetic background; perhaps even in the United States and Canada. With the figures for the white population in general the same as for Australia (phenotypic expression might also be expected to be similar since both countries have a high rate of red meat consumption), the proportion of **carriers** in the Afrikaner population is nearly one in six; and when the calculations are based on **males only, one in five.** From the study it was inferred that the HH gene had already attained its high frequency in the populations of Holland, Germany and France before 1652, the year in which the European settlement at the Cape began, and that it was introduced into the local population by a number of persons at different times.

In this case, every community elswhere, with a population which is predominantly Dutch, French or German could manifest the same gene rate.

The high frequency of the Hemochromatosis gene, wherever it occurs, has been attributed to Darwinian selection.[vii] In an environment poor in available iron and frequently infested with internal parasites, the Hemochromatosis gene would have been decidedly protective against the adverse effect of iron deficiency in early humans. The gene continues to flourish today because the devastating effects of excessive iron loading do not appear until well beyond the reproductive years.[iii]

There are experts who believe that Hemochromatosis may prove to be the scourge of the 21st century if responsible governments do not take steps now to combat it. With an estimated 2.5 million carriers in Canada and nearly 32 million in the United States, for instance, the situation can surely only compound itself. **"If the potentially lethal iron loading gene is as prevalent as the current evidence suggests,"** say the South Africans, and in so doing concur with what experts in several countries are saying, **"then concerted attempts should be made in epidemiological surveys to identify asymptomatic homozygotes by applying screening tests with a high sensitivity and predictive accuracy.**[xiv]**"**

One does not "catch" HH; one inherits it. It is not one of those genetic legacies which deters one from having children. Once it has been established that parents are carriers, their offspring can be monitored and prophylactically treated to prevent the accumulation of excess iron. Furthermore, individuals who are made aware early in life that dietary intake of iron can accelerate the iron loading, would certainly avoid the use of supplements.

What this means to us

To accentuate the hypotheses, among the 600 athletes who represented Canada at the Los Angeles Olympics, **nearly 80** could be "heterozygotes" for Hemochromatosis; in other words carriers of the recessive gene which, when two heterozygotes marry, will be responsible for producing children who will be at risk from a disease which will cause them to accumulate iron from every conceivable source. **Two out of four children will** in turn, be **carriers**, but the genetic make-up of **one out of four** of the offspring will be such that, unless steps are taken to prevent the ravages, they **may develop the full-blown disease.** These are mathematically estimated averages. I know of a family of nine, in which all nine members are afflicted.

It was extremely interesting to learn from the Canadian study that there were some clinical manifestations in carriers too: arthralgia, or joint disease, (19%), diabetes (3%) and prominent skin pigmentation (2%). Liver enzymes were elevated in 13%. A similar proportion of normal subjects had these manifestations; however, two members of the Canadian Hemochromatosis Society who presented with most of the involvements of the full-blown disease, were found to carry only a single gene.

Working on conservative figures of 10%-13% and one person in three-hundred, respectively, in one capacity seating of Vancouver's B.C. Place Stadium there could be between 6,000 and 7,800 carriers and approximately 200 of those present would already be under treatment for, or could—if not detected in time— suffer from diabetes, arthritis, cardiac problems or cirrhosis of the liver. Again, due to a lack of statistics for other ethnic groups, it should be pointed out that this number would only apply to a totally Caucasian attendance. No cases of hereditary Hemochromatosis have been discovered among the Native Indian people or the Inuit.

Although the groups which have been selected to illustrate the point may not, themselves, necessarily be representative of Canada as a whole, they serve to underline a situation which deserves to be brought to the notice of anyone who is not aware of the existence of this insiduous killer. Certainly, in British Columbia to the estimated 10,000 affected individuals, and the 286,320 who could be carriers of one gene for HH. (Creighton S, Hayden M. Hemochromatosis in B.C. B.C.M.J. 1984; 26:613-4)

Every year millions of dollars are being spent by the various Provincial health care systems in the treatment of diseases which are actually only the end result of a disorder which renders the human body incapable of ridding itself of excess iron. Unless the underlying cause is diagnosed and the correct therapy instituted, much of the expenditure will prove to have been in vain. The fatal complications can never be alleviated without the removal of the stored iron; if that is not done, the prognosis is hopeless. Furthermore, since only the immediate cause of death will appear on the death certificate, future generations will be not be forewarned.

At this moment there must be thousands who, if they have Hemochromatosis, are experiencing inexplicable bouts of weakness or fatigue; many (who appear extraordinarily healthy because of it) will be more delighted than concerned about a tan which persists long after the summer has passed; in every corner of this country, there are men who are secretly terrified because incidents which seem to threaten the very essence of their maleness, are becoming the rule rather than the exception. Stiffness and pains in some of the joints will be dismissed, by the young of both sexes, as belonging to old age and therefore transient—until, one day, they find that the once fleeting discomfort is now persistent and has become a constant agony.

Then, the passing of time will bring, perhaps, the first signs of sudden or maturity-onset diabetes which might grow progressively more resistant to insulin. By this time, the male victim might have become concerned about the fact that he seems to have less hair on his chest and his legs are as smooth as a woman's; he is losing his eyelashes . In common with many female sufferers from the disorder, he finds that his memory seems to be failing; he has periods of extreme confusion, is depressed and is frequently irritable to the point of being downright quarrelsome.

His wife—who is beside herself because she can find no explanation for his lack of interest in her—concludes that he must be having an affair but dares not question him because experience has taught her that he will fly into a rage. Worse still, if she is sexually active and has concluded, as one woman wrote, that her husband is "over the hill", she may seek solace elsewhere. Meanwhile our hypothetical victim should be going easy on liquor, should, in fact be avoiding red wine altogether, and would be advised to take tea with his morning egg instead of orange juice.[xi;xii] At this stage, a liver biopsy might show that he has micro nodular cirrhosis, or worse.

The picture I have painted might be extreme but it is by no means as rare as one would suppose. I have been told of several cases which parallel this. It is, more often than not, the wives who write, and I can identify with the ones who describe how they resorted, in vain, to tinting their hair, going on a diet and splurging on a new wardrobe.

Those Hemochromatotics who are fortunate, may be correctly diagnosed by an astute physician before too much tissue damage occurs. Others, who, tragically, are in the majority, will go from doctor to doctor, disillusioned because none of those consulted over a period of years has been able to explain years and years of nagging abdominal pain or bouts of nausea; let alone the reason why hair which was once the pride and joy of its owner has lost its texture, has become as fine as a baby's and is now of indeterminate colour. To make matters worse, the once magnificent tan is now a sickly, slate grey. "I was desperate enough to consult a witch-doctor," was what an Ontario woman confessed, after what seemed to her to have been an eternity of ill-health.

Iron Supplements

Prompted by commercials depicting the glow of youth and the physical well-being promised by the media, many of these desperate people will resort to vitamins and, for them, **iron supplements could prove fatal!**

While conceding that iron deficiency still exists in certain areas of the population, there is some concern about the type of advertising which has led the public to the belief that iron supplements are a "cure-all" for everything from senility to impotence. There is the alarming prospect of people relying upon self-diagnosis and self-prescription of iron without their having been warned of some of the possible consequences of its use. Such symptoms as fatigue, lethargy, dizziness and loss of memory could as much be signs of iron overload as of iron deficiency.

There appears to be a tremendous lack of responsibility on the part of sports writers and other individuals who promote iron as the key to performance, health and beauty, without modifying their statements. The very expression to "pump iron" suggests a connection between the mineral and strength, and an article which appeared in a travel magazine some months ago, under this seemingly innocuous heading, went as far as to suggest that there is no-one who will not benefit from supplementation. Another story which featured an interview with a doctor of sports medicine at the University of British Columbia, brought a spate of protest from Hemochromatotics.

The doctor had apparently stated, according to the article, that an iron supplement was the only realistic treatment for a condition which is characterized by "a definite lack of performance, frequent injury and fatigue". Most of those who voiced concern, did so on the grounds that, since there was already a temptation among some sportsmen to resort to steroids, there was a grave risk attached to suggesting that the intake of iron would magically change an under-performing athlete into an Olympic star. And when telephoned, the doctor in question was in complete agreement. He would never dream, was his assurance, of prescribing iron for anyone **without preliminary tests**!

"The diagnosis of Hemochromatosis is easy," writes William H. Crosby, M.D. "It requires the demonstration of increased amounts of iron." (Arch Intern Med—Vol 146, June 1986)

In more than one centre, medical societies have passed resolutions to have government agencies consider making it mandatory for over-the-counter iron pills and dietary iron supplements, to carry a warning label stating that chronic daily use of extra iron is a hazard to individuals with HH. The Canadian Hemochromatosis Society has written in the same vein, on several occasions, to the Federal Minister of Health. Early in April, 1988, a direct request to this effect was submitted to the Hon. Peter Dueck, Minister of Health for British Columbia; a request which I repeated in person when I was privileged to meet with Premier Bill vander Zalm on April 22, 1988.

Cancer and Excess Iron

"For some people iron is a carcinogen,"states the writer of an article in "Ironic Blood", newsletter of the Iron Overload Diseases Association Inc., in the March-April 1988 edition which is dedicated to the American College of Physicians. "If not you, if not a member of your family, someone you know has the genetic make-up that causes storage of excess iron. The metabolic abnormality is estimated in one out of 200 people."

The relationship of cancer to excess iron has been studied at Indiana University. Eugene D. Weinberg, M.D.,quoted a study showing that in 20 humans with breast cancer, the tissue contained 3 times as much iron as normal breast tissue. (P.M. Santoliquido, H.W. Southwick and J.H. Olwin, Surg. Gyn. Obstet. 142,65; 1976) In another study, 88% of breast cancer patients tested with high serum ferritin. (R.C. Coombs, T.J. Poules and J.C. Gazet, Cancer 40, 937, 1977.)

Iron In Our Food

It is impossible to maintain an iron-free diet. Every cereal contains iron. All wheat products are routinely fortified and, to make matters worse, many manufacturers add extra iron—which sells the product to more people. Only people who are faced with the dilemma of eliminating iron could sympathize with the woman who, overjoyed at finding cookies which were evidently safe for her husband to eat because they were "iron reduced", had to discover that what the label did, in fact, state was that the product contained "reduced iron." She was feeding him iron in a form which is more readily assimilated!

In March, 1978, the American publication, Medical Tribune, quoted a warning expressed by the prominent Swedish researcher, Dr. K.S. Olsson, that "the iron project" (referring to what they termed the 'beefing up' of iron levels in bread and other flour products) would necessitate a new vigilance on the part of doctors for the disorder (Hemochromatosis) in males. He claimed first-hand knowledge since he had seen the "rare" genetic condition surface in his own country only after Sweden had approved adding iron to bread about 30 years before.

"Now you hardly ever see an iron deficiency anemia," he said. "What you do see, instead, are a number of patients with too much iron."

Not even Doctor Olssen could have foreseen the extent to

which the disorder would surface. He certainly could not have expected that, far from only requiring vigilance for iron overload in males, women could be afflicted to the extent which today has proved to be the case; nor could he have imagined that, within a short period, that country, Sweden, would see a case involving an eleven year-old girl with diabetes and disease of the heart muscle from Hemochromatosis.[xiii]

Tea and Orange Juice

There is ample evidence that absorption of iron from individual food items is profoundly affected by the composition of the meal as a whole. For example, egg iron is very poorly absorbed, but the percentage of absorption is greatly increased by drinking orange juice with it.[xii]

HH patients are thus advised to take their orange juice between meals, as vitamin C, even in low doses, increases the absorption of iron from food.

The interest in tea was aroused during a study of the absorption of iron from cornmeal porridge served with sugar containing ferrous sulphate and ascorbic acid. When tea was drunk with the meal, the absorption seemed lower than was expected.[xi]

To a Hemochromatotic, Vitamin C can be harmful.

It is not suggested that HH people **avoid** vitamin C, because studies have shown that iron-overloaded people are deficient in that vitamin. All that is required is common sense.

It is important to note that larger doses, 500-1000 mg. or more, may, in addition, cause a redistribution of iron in the body from one organ, such as the liver, to another, such as the heart, which may precipitate serious heart problems.

In the same way that certain foods work against one another, some food elements work together. One trace element which works **against iron,** is ZINC. "If you're iron overloaded, you're likely to be zinc deficient," says Stanley Skoryna, MD., PhD., Director of the Gastrointestinal Research Laboratory at McGill University in Montreal. He suggests that HH patients emphasize foods high in zinc to help block iron absorption.

McGraw-Hills's 1979 revised edition of Nutrition Almanac

says:"... Excessive intake of zinc may result in a loss of iron and copper from the liver.... ..... a diabetic pancreas contains only about half as much zinc as a healthy one. ... Zinc is beneficial to the diabetic because of its regulatory effect on insulin in the blood."

N.B. Hemochromatosis is also spelt "Haemochromatosis". The spelling used in this book is that which is in common use in North America.

CHAPTER TWO

The Disease

HEMOCHROMATOSIS, WHICH IS CAUSED BY AN OVERLOAD of iron in the body, is primarily an hereditary condition; an "inborn error of metabolism".[iv] The disease (which, in itself is many diseases) has also been known to develop as a result of long standing dietary intake in sufficient quantity, alcohol excess, multiple transfusions and other causes, all of which would come under the heading of secondary Hemochromatosis. There are, for instance, many recorded cases of iron-overload disease among black people in South Africa, with no genetic defect, who cook and brew beer in iron drums and prefer to cook in iron pots. My family and I knew such a person very well, as I have described in one of my books, but the work I have chosen to do, concerns, for the most part, victims of the hereditary form of the disorder.

Once the excess iron lodges in a vital organ, damaging or even destroying it, it causes much suffering, frequently in the form of diabetes which is often resistant to insulin; and when the skin takes on the characteristic colour (in some cases, a "tan which never fades"; in others, a slate grey), this is commonly referred to as "Bronze Diabetes". Symptoms vary, but many Hemochromatotics experience chronic fatigue, severe abdominal pain, bouts of nausea, diminished memory and disorientation for many years before diagnosis. In later years there could be some degree of hearing loss. The disease is frequently misdiagnosed as chronic hepatitis, sudden-onset diabetes, etc.. One of the earliest symptoms is arthritis of the knuckles of the first and second fingers.

The liver, heart, endocrine glands (glands of internal secretion, such as the pancreas), skin and joints are principally affected, and cirrhosis, cardiomyopathy (disease of the heart muscle), diabetes mellitus, hypogonadism (deficient activity of testis or ovary) and arthritis, are the usual manifestations.[viii] By the time clinical manifestations appear,—in other words signs that have become sufficiently evident for the examining physician to detect them—iron overload is eventually fatal unless the iron is eliminated.

The common causes of death are cardiac failure, arrhythmia (irregularity in the beating of the heart), hepatic (liver) failure, hepatoma (tumour of the liver) or other malignancy, or the complications of diabetes.[viii] Before the advent of insulin, diabetes topped the list. Formerly, when the diagnosis was made **clinically**, cirrhosis and skin pigmentation were almost always present; often accompanied by diabetes mellitus, hypogonadism (diminished sexual function) arthritis and cardiac failure. Today the picture is changing, as diagnostic methods improve.

Victims who are not discovered soon enough may develop cancer of the liver; ''hence the importance of family screening and early treatment of affected individuals cannot be emphasized too strongly''. . . . (1) All first-degree relatives over the age of ten years should be investigated. (2) Tests for serum iron concentration, percentage saturation of transferrin and serum ferritin concentration should be performed. (3) When screening tests are equivocal, successive investigations over a number of years are recommended.[v] Until recently it was considered safe to limit serial investigation to individuals who are eighteen and older. However, I was informed recently by the Dean of Medicine, that the age had been lowered from eighteen to twelve, at the University of Western Ontario.

Perhaps one of the most tragic effects is that of testicular atrophy, which is present in about 25% of male patients.[viii]. Loss of libido may often antedate the other clinical manifestations of the disease.[v] It seems that diminished sexual function is a relatively frequent finding in young subjects; men of all ages appear to experience this, however.

I did not realise that this was the case, until the first letter I received in which my correspondent confided ''my sex life has gone to hell!'', was followed by numerous others, worded differently but expressing the same sentiment. The loss of body hair, which all who suffer this find so distressing, is related and is due to pituitary involvement. Usually the hair grows back to some extent after removal of storage iron, but it is scanty. I have seen men, after nearly ten years of therapy, with hairless legs and hardly more than fluff on the chest.

Women, too, can be affected by hypogonadism, as manifested by secondary amenorrhea (absence or abnormal interruption of the menstrual flow) diminished libido and loss of sexual hair. Of course, there are many causes of amenorrhea, Hemochromatosis being one of the least common, but iron deposited in the pituitary gland does impair the production of sex hormones. The young woman who contacted me because she was so deeply afraid that she would never have children, was one of the motivating forces in the founding of the Hemochromatosis society— although she may never know this. Not only was she a homozygote for Hemochromatosis; she had been treated with iron supplements.

Unfortunately, many authors of books on nutrition and dietary supplements do not appear to take this menace seriously. Some dismiss it quite airily and those who do have some knowledge of the disease as it is manifested in the form of "Bronze Diabetes" or "Pigmented Cirrhosis", are not often acquainted, for example, with the type of arthritis caused by the accumulation of excessive iron..

It is interesting to note that the prevalence and severity of the iron overload which is so common in the South African black population is declining in urban areas as a result of changing drinking patterns.[xiv]

As commercially manufactured beer, brewed in stainless steel, replaces the traditional home brew to the benefit of the black, the white population on the other hand are running the risk of "Potjiekos Peril." This is the title of an article featured in Personality Magazine, and refers to the current penchant for "potjiekos"—a stew simmered over the coals in a three-legged iron pot, which is as much part of a barbeque as steak and chops. The Falconbridge Iron Foundry stands to make a million with the introduction of the first, rustproof "potjie". It will probably also be contributing to a reduction in the intake of iron, without realizing that in, so doing, it is performing a public service.

I feel that I should, perhaps, apologize to those members of the medical profession who are supportive of my efforts but considerably irritated by the way many of us loosely refer to HH as "the bronze killer". However, I excuse the selection of this title for my book on the grounds that, if I was not aware at the time I started writing, that there was more to Hemochromatosis than diabetes coupled with a mahogany-coloured skin— and that all the other complications were a **part** of it and not merely co-incidental I had encountered many physicians who did not know this either. There are still doctors who insist that the disease is too rare to warrant serious concern. Other serious misconceptions are that the disease only afflicts men in their middle years— or older—and that women are not affected; if they are, it is the popular belief that HH will strike only after the menopause or a hysterectomy.

The files of the Canadian Hemochromatosis Society tell a different story; a tragic story. Those who have been diagnosed in time are overwhelmingly grateful to the researchers who labour unceasingly, and strive towards greater understanding, earlier diagnosis and a happier prognosis for those who are afflicted. "The frequency of Hemochromatosis is unquestionably underestimated because the diagnosis in the past was restricted to the end stage of the disease, and not always made even then," stated Corwin Q. Edwards et al as long ago as 1977.[vi] (Diagnosis in Siblings and Children: New England Journal of Medicine.) And now it is thought that in some countries as many as 16% of the Caucasian are carriers of the recessive gene!

While it is true that, **on an average**, women become symptomatic later than their male counterparts, there is the recorded death at seventeen of a young girl on the lower mainland of British Columbia. There has been previous reference to the eleven year old Swedish girl with diabetes and disease of the heart muscle[xiii]. In the next chapter, mention is made of two little sisters on phlebotomy therapy in Vancouver.

A charter member of the Canadian Hemochromatosis society reports that she suffered from stiff, painful joints at 21; by the time she was finally diagnosed, more than ten years later (when her brother became seriously ill) her transferrin saturation was 99%. . . . twice the upper limit of normal! The brother's history confounds most of the generally accepted statistics: Hemochromatosis was further advanced in his early thirties than my husband's was at 50. Neither of the parents had exhibited any of the symptoms.

My own daughter was diagnosed at 32, and it is only because she was was blessed to have a family doctor who—knowing her father's history—agreed to have her tested purely on the grounds that she was tired and just didn't "feel right", that she has suffered no damage to her liver. A normal transferrin saturation for a young woman of her age might have been in the region of 25%. Hers was 95%!

Phlebotomy Therapy

There is no cure for Hemochromatosis; treatment is ongoing, for life—and the pun is intended. But, especially when detected early, a series of phlebotomies or " blood-lettings" (venesection is another term used to describe the procedure) can greatly reduce the build-up of excess iron in the body, thus alleviating many of the complications. Removal of the iron prolongs survival, cures the cardiomyopathy and the skin pigmentation, and arrests the liver damage. Diabetes may improve, but hypogonadism and arthropathy do not, and hepatoma may develop even years later,[viii] if the liver disease is far advanced.

To those who suffer these ravages, the true tragedy of this disease lies in the fact that the hypogonadism and cirrhosis, when related to Hemochromatosis **were preventable**. The suffering was unnecessary. If subsequent generations are checked, and iron loading prevented, they will be spared much.

There are a few patients who, after the commencement of phlebotomy therapy, experience an initial aggravation of symptoms, particularly those which involve the heart; some say that they are affected with severe leg cramps and joint pains for some days after being bled. However, the benefits far outweigh the discomfort. I recall the expression used by the legendary Professor Thomas Bothwell of South Africa, and most people report having indeed enjoyed that feeling of "increased well-being" once phlebotomy therapy was commenced. My husband described it as a "lightening of the body and spirit."

It must be remembered that, once the disease is advanced, it is an **awful** amount of blood which has to be taken from these people! Since it is the "Gee whiz items" which make people sit up and take notice, I inevitably mention what is involved in phlebotomy therapy, when I am interviewed by the media, and it never fails.

"WHAT? A GALLON OF BLOOD A MONTH! You must be joking!"

But this is no joke; not for the doctor who has to make himself available, possibly twice a week over a long period, and certainly not for the patient who knows that it could take two years or more before the desired elimination of storage iron is achieved. Phlebotomy leads to a marked increase in iron absorption. If the treatment is stopped, the serum iron level and percentage saturation of transferrin promptly increase and precede the increase in serum ferritin concentration. **Iron stores reaccumulate**; thus it is important to emphasize that **lifelong phlebotomy therapy is required, preferably on a regular, rather than an intermittent basis.**[v]

Letters reflect a wide variety of concerns. A retired R.C.M.P. officer wonders whether it is correct that the hospital charges a user fee every time he goes there for his bleed; when patients require two venesections a week, the cost, in any five-week month, could amount to $100. "I'm sick of the whole, bloody business!" wails a Saskatchewan housewife, while the most common complaint is that, while the extracted blood is used for plasma in some countries, in Canada—because the Red Cross will not use even that which is taken from the young, potential victim as a prophylactic or preventative measure—it has been known to end up as fertilizer for the physician's roses!

Almost everyone reports difficult periods when "they couldn't get the blood out of me last time!" or "no-one takes my bleed seriously." "Last week I waited for hours in emergency while every sore toe was given preference!" Many patients are, however, treated at a hospital by their own physicians, at a prearranged time, which is not always as satisfactory an arrangement as it may appear. Frequently the doctor in question is the specialist who diagnosed the disorder and is happy to undertake treatment of the complications; but he does not necessarily want to be involved for years and years in the venesection part of it.

The most commonly expressed concern is about the frequency with which further treatment should be carried out. There is comfort to be derived from the fact that, once the desired level has been achieved, three to four phlebotomies a year should suffice. But it cannot be stressed too strongly that (a) to reduce the stored iron to that extent, may take several years and (b) it should not be left to the physician to take the first steps in initiating the follow-up therapy. This is a critical stage and it is in the interest of every Hemochromatotic to ensure that regular tests are carried out. Naturally there are those for whom, at the time of diagnosis, it was already too late, but I prefer to quote Bassett, Halliday and Powell. "The patient can be reassured that the prognosis is excellent, provided that iron re-accumulation does not occur over the long period of follow-up."[v]

Sure, it **is** a "bloody business" and it is understandable that anyone would grow heartily sick of it, but all accept the fact that they will not stay alive without it. No matter how depressed the person is at the prospect of having to regard this as part of the rest of his or her life, the first phlebotomy is the first step on the road to hope. All Hemochromatotics who undergo this form of therapy owe their lives to Professor C.A. Finch of Seattle, who first instituted therapeutic phlebotomy.[ix] One could go back further: to Bothwell and Edwards and Charlton and Powell, and Canada's own Valberg; to Jacobs and Bassett and Halliday and Cook; and on. . . . and on. . . . back to those who have been doing research and writing about it since 1865.

If the iron is not removed, the 5-year survival rate after diagnosis is 18%, and the 10-year survival rate, 6%.[viii]

Treatment should never be suspended or the frequency of phlebotomies decreased because of difficult bleedings. Quoted in "Ironic Blood", Dr. Barry Skikne maintains that it is unnecessary to have a phlebotomy by the usual techniques of a vacuum bag and a large guage needle.

Phlebotomists at the University of Kansas use 19, or even 21-guage needles with scalp-vein; otherwise known as a butterfly needle. The blood is withdrawn slowly by two large syringes, 60cc, without much damage to the vein.

It usually takes about 20 minutes, which is not much longer than the usual method.

In cases where 500cc is not tolerated, the size of the unit to be removed can be adjusted. All problems have been avoided since this method was started, Dr. Skikne says.

He advises patients to drink plenty of fluids before and after phlebotomies. In cases of low blood pressure or extreme dizziness, a saline solution can be given to replace fluids.

CHAPTER THREE

How do I know if I have it?''

ONE OF THE AIMS OF THE CANADIAN HEMOCHROMATOSIS Society, which was established in 1982, is to stimulate awareness among practising physicians and members of the public so that potential victims may be diagnosed in time. When the disease is considered to be hereditary, the sufferer is immediately counselled to have his or her family screened, serum transferrin saturation and serum ferritin being the best screening tests for HH. If one or both tests are abnormal, further tests can be done to establish the degree of iron loading. These tests include the demonstration of iron in a liver biopsy specimen, measurement of liver density with computed tomography (CT scan), or—where available—Magnetic Resonance Imaging (MRI).

In families where the HLA (Histocompatability leukocyte antigens) haplotypes of a homozygote are known, determination of the HLA—A and B haplotypes of relatives may be used to identify other family members at risk of developing iron overload. HLA, otherwise known as tissue typing, is usually reserved for families in which the results of the transferrin and serum ferritin are inconclusive; where blood loss, for some reason, or iron therapy make the interpretation of these tests difficult.

HLA typing is particularly helpful in identifying homozygotes at risk of iron overload in families where there has been a homozygous-heterozygous mating—which proved to be the case in my own family. Unfortunately, however, HLA typing is a privilege which is not readily available in too many centres in Canada and, even where it is, government funding, in some instances, has been reduced.

There was a time when one of the main problems in this regard was the fact that geneticists are generally more involved in pediatric rather than adult genetics; however, it now seems that pediatricians will have to become increasingly involved in the genetics and treatment of HH.

When the Hemochromatosis Research Foundation featured a photograph of Benji Palmer of California in ''Hemochromatosis Awareness'', it was thought that, at the age of 7 1/2, Benji was the youngest HH patient in the world on phlebotomy therapy. That is, however, not the the case. Last year, after liver biopsies had established the diagnosis, three young children—two little girls and their brother—whose ages ranged from 3 to 7 years of age, commenced treatment at the children's hospital in Vancouver, British Columbia; the 7-year-old girl already manifesting some liver damage. There are recorded cases of severe iron overload in even younger children. HH is no longer a disease of just the mature.

The diagnosis of homozygotes in the Canadian study[iii] was made by determining the number of persons with a transferrin saturation of more than 55%, and an abnormally high serum ferritin measurement. When the accuracy of biochemical methods was assessed by discriminant function analysis, the correct classification rate, using transferrin saturation alone in predicting whether people are homozygotes—without HLA typing —was 98.3%, and only slightly higher using transferrin saturation combined with tests for high ferritin levels.

In this study, conducted at the University of Western Ontario, and involving men and women between the ages of 21 and 78, clinical data was obtained by looking specifically for joint pain and stiffness, skin pigmentation, diabetes, hepatomegaly (enlarged liver) and heart failure. The most common symptom was that of joint pain and stiffness—which was manifested by 59% of homozygotes. 56% had enlarged livers, 31% were diabetic, 30% had some degree of skin pigmentation, there was some enlargement of the heart in 11% and the figure for heart failure was 11%.

A further 15% had no symptoms at the time of diagnosis and one wonders what their fate would have been, had they not been detected in this manner.

It struck me as significant that both men and women were tested and that young people were included; but what is astounding is the fact that so few medical practitioners are aware that research of this kind is being undertaken in Canada. Doctor Leslie Valberg, then Professor of Medicine at the university at which the study was carried out, has been engaged in Hemochromatosis research for more than twenty years. He is a highly respected authority and I am exceedingly grateful to him for his patient and clear replies to the endless questions with which I constantly bombard him.

So much is known now; so much has been done; what a shame that the benefits of research take so long to filter through to the ones who need them most. Far too frequently, concerned families find that it is one thing to be told what is recommended, and quite another matter altogether to find, readily, (a) a doctor who will requisition for it and (b) a laboratory where someone knows what is required. It is not uncommon to be told that the blood ''needs to be sent to the States!'' or, ''your hemoglobin is normal'' or, most erroneous of all, ''if there was anything wrong, it would have shown up in some other blood tests!''

The reason for carrying out, particularly, a blood test for plasma transferrin saturation **combined** with one for plasma ferritin is that, in families of known sufferers (the latter are referred to as ''probands'') these will provide sensitive indices of Hemochromatosis. For the benefit of anyone who is having problems obtaining the correct tests, I wish to pass on what I learned from Professor Valberg: that plasma iron fluctuates and, by itself, is not a good index of iron loading; the ratio of plasma iron to the iron binding protein, transferrin, is known to be a better indicator of the disordered iron metabolism in the disease. Hemoglobin, which is the oxygen-carrying pigment of the blood, is normal in HH —except in rare cases—but is monitored during prolonged phlebotomy therapy so that, if the level drops too low, bleeding may be halted for a period.

It is doubtful whether relatives of diagnosed individuals are always given the correct blood tests to determine whether or not they are at risk; nor can there be too much confidence in the standard of treatment in some areas. There are instances where the patient, having been diagnosed in one city, returns to a another where treatment is in the hands of different practitioners who do not—as one woman put it—"know how the levels tie in." In the survey carried out early this year by the CHS, only two people knew what tests their physicians utilized in determining the frequency of phlebotomies.

No sensible Hemochromatotic patient readily moves from one place to another without first establishing whether therapy and monitoring of his or her condition can be maintained in the new environment. Because it is frequently called upon to find a knowledgeable family practitioner in a particular area, the CHS has been obliged to operate a doctor referral service.

CHAPTER FOUR

Significant signs

I THINK I MAY BE FORGIVEN FOR MY CONTINUED PREOCCU-pation with the "bronze" aspect of this killer. Several studies have been conducted in which no cases of such pigmentation were detected, but I have encountered very few Hemochromatotics without **some** degree of bronzing. Because of our own experience, I had always believed that everyone who had this hyperpigmentation would look like an advertisement for the beach at Waikiki. However, it is sometimes present as little more than brown patches in various parts of the body; for example the small of the back or high up the legs, just below the buttocks; from ankles to calves; the top of the foot, between toes and ankles.

"I am really not sure of the chronology leading towards the recognition of Hemochromatosis," writes George H. of Willowdale, Ontario. "About 1978 I noticed a feeling of tiredness and general lethargy, although my wife claims she was aware of it developing three or four years earlier. As a result I joined a fitness club because I thought that poor physical condition and advancing years were the culprits. By then I noticed my tan, for whatever reason, seemed to be best on my lower legs. . . . I used to lie under the sunning lamps at the fitness club to help my tan become more uniform. . . .

"My ashen colour developed gradually. I didn't particularly notice but I was shocked at how old I looked in photographs. Even my mother, then in her mid 70's, once told me that something must be wrong, because the way I looked, she was going to outlive me!''

Having read that the colour is prominent around old scars, I expected that the marks, themselves, would always show up bronze, but found that the scar sometimes appears white in contrast to the deep mahogany colour of the skin immediately surrounding it. I have since learned that the colour is dependent upon whether the cicatrix was forming during the period of iron loading or before. When obliging gentlemen roll up trouser legs to show me, the skin thus exhibited is frequently dry and scaly—like old sunburn ready to rub off.

Don of Victoria recalls that flaking of the skin on his shins commenced way back, at the same time as he discovered that he had diabetes. Arthritis had manifested itself some six years before. A month after the diagnosis of diabetes, he picked up a germ (?) virus (?) amoeba (?) in Europe. The cause of this sickness was never isolated, but it was serious enough to land him in hospital, in isolation and on the critical list, for a month. He was off work for seven months and, although he only weighed 155 lbs to begin with, he lost a further 25. Whatever it was that had incapacitated him is not known to be related to HH; but it seems to prove that, however many blood samples are taken, iron overload does not show up unless specific tests are done.

In 1981, eight years after the first, clinical symptoms had appeared, cirrhosis of the liver—together with bronzing of the skin and all the other involvements—led to a diagnosis of Hemochromatosis. Initially half a litre of blood was extracted, per week, and a year later he could say that he seemed to feel better and that the skin flaking had been reduced. It is evident from looking at him, that his joints remain very painful and he has periods of great fatigue.

The first sign noticed by Bill, also of Victoria, was that the skin on his legs "went funny". As British as they come, he describes recurrent lumps which appeared under his arm and which were removed; but none of the doctors to whom I have spoken seem to link them with HH. What seems most significant is that, as was the case with Don, iron overload again was not detected in tests carried out before surgery. He was driven by severe arthritic pain to consult his doctor again, and, this time, because the latter was away on holiday, was seen by the doctor's partner. He—according to Bill—"knew at once what was wrong." After five years of venesection therapy, Bill is still deeply pigmented, a borderline diabetic and another who talks wryly about his blood "going on the roses!" When I last spoke to him, there had been little improvement in his condition but he is comforted by the fact that there has also been no deterioration—which would have been the case without blood removal. He is one of hundreds who are plagued with leg cramps.

* * *

It is interesting to note that the bronzing is not due to iron in the bloodstream, as so many people assume. This degree of pigmentation is caused by melanin and while, in the early stage, it can be attractive and lend the patient a healthy appearance, it can be misleading and deprive the victim of much-needed sympathy. By the time the discolouration is due to actual iron, it has become an unhealthy and unattractive slate grey. Some degree of discolouration is a natural part of the aging process, but it can become evident in Hemochromatotics both young and old; when it appears in conjunction with other symptoms, it deserves attention.

If the area in which pigmentation occurs is in a part of the body normally exposed to the sun, one could take the cause for granted, as Helen C. of Vancouver did. She had been aware of brown patches on her arms for five years but was quite unconcerned —despite the fact that she had been distressingly fatigued during this period, suffered from high blood pressure, has a sister, Grace, who had been under treatment for Hemochromatosis for some time, and a brother who died of cirrhosis of the liver. Their mother died of diabetes. In addition to crippling pain in her muscles and joints, Helen was plagued with bad headaches and recurrent spells of weakness.

It was Grace's dentist who made the discovery that her iron levels were high and, for this, she is grateful; but how much Helen could have been spared if timely HLA typing or transferrin saturation tests had established that she was a homozygote, when her sister was first diagnosed! Curiously, Grace is one of several people whose iron overload was first recognised by a dentist. I do not, however, have the necessary authorization to recount their histories.

That anyone can go for years with rust-coloured ankles without seeking a reason for this, may seem extraordinary, but it happens. Because his hemoglobin was high, M.S. of Richmond was, quite correctly, said to be suffering from polycythemia—a condition in which there is an excess of red corpuscles in the blood. This could be caused, for instance, by smoking, but could be quite normal among people who live at very high altitudes where there is less oxygen in the air. M.S. has a family history of heart disease; his father and brother both died at 50. Tests showed high triglycerides, and other symptoms included tiredness, weight loss, disorientation and periodic bouts of depression.

The credit for his diagnosis must go to his wife.

In 1983, on reading an account of an interview with me, written by Tom Fletcher in the Richmond Review, she was immediately struck by a reference to "rusty ankles" and, although it took courage to do so, requested that her husband be tested for HH. They are blessed with a doctor who keeps an open mind and Mr. S. has been on a course of phlebotomies ever since. As beforesaid, Hemoglobin is very rarely high in Hemochromatosis, and when other signs point to an excess of iron, the reason for this polycythemia should be very thoroughly investigated. Mrs. S. says her husband is able to think very much more clearly than before embarking on the therapy. Perhaps the time will come when physicians will be quick to investigate the phenomena of hyperpigmentation, no matter what the cause may be.

Tom Fletcher was also responsible for saddling me with the title of "Richmond's Iron Lady"—a title which takes too much living up to. His article, which was more widely read than its writer knew, brought responses from people in many parts of the lower mainland, one of them being D.D. who not only told me a very interesting case history but agreed to be filmed for television while undergoing a phlebotomy. That story, with the kind co-operation of D's doctor and the staff of the Royal Columbian Hospital in New Westminster, B.C., subsequently appeared on the news service of VU 13. It generated a further response from Hemochromatotics—and a conversation with the doctor conccrried, led me to Dr. Valberg, who, to our very great joy, is now the chief medical adviser to the Canadian Hemochromatosis Society.

D.D. had been having problems for nine years, since the age of 31. He recalls having a "very low energy level" and being constantly tired. There were times when he suffered from such intense pain in the area of the liver that he was off work once for three months. He was told that he had chronic hepatitis and it was not until he consulted the physician who later appeared with him on television, that Hemochromatosis was diagnosed. A liver biopsy confirmed the doctor's diagnosis and plebotomies twice weekly were initiated. At the age of forty, he still had not regained much energy but the fatigue had become less constant.

Athletes and Arthritis

Many I have interviewed, report having spent a great deal of time outdoors, but an aversion to heat and ultraviolet light becomes very common later; skin problems sometimes result from exposure. A significant number have been swimmers, runners, enthusiastic gardeners; and this makes one wonder whether the fact that Hemochromatotics so frequently have been athletic, energetic to a marked degree and endowed with exceptional physical strength, is due to their special make-up or is simply a remarkable coincidence.

Maureen W. tells me that, before she started complaining that she was too tired, she had been a competitive swimmer for seven years and was involved in Little Theatre and the Outboard Club; she did heavy gardening—"like stump-pulling by hand"—and was extremely fit. Pain and stiffness were attributed to over-use of the affected joints. Then, at age 21, "I just did not feel myself," she says. "At first they put this down to the aftermath of a virus 'flu; then to 'female frustrations'. . . . The symptoms are so vague until the damage has been done!"

Don had been a sprinter; my Tom might have swum in the Olympics. T.R. of Sidney, B.C. used to do a great deal of racing in small sailing boats, some of which have a trapeze. This demands a high degree of agility because, as he explains: "You go out on the end of the trapeze using rapid knee movements." He was in Mauritius, in his early forties, when he found that he was getting too stiff to do this and concluded that ''old age was creeping up'' on him.

From Mauritius, he moved to Australia where, two years later, he began to be troubled with stiff, sore feet in the mornings. A local doctor told him: ''At your age you probably have arthritis.'' Drugs were prescribed which ''seemed to be of help and things eased off a bit.'' Then, about eleven or twelve years ago, the pain became really bad; it was there ''all the time . . . every day!''

He saw many different doctors over a period until, eventually he ''got fed up!'' Someone suggested he go to an arthritic clinic and he went to the Royal Prince Alfred Hospital in Sydney, Australia, where it was soon decided that his problem was not straight-forward arthritis. Further tests showed iron overload. He says that it was lucky for him that, at that clinic, they knew about Hemochromatosis and referred him to a physician who was treating several patients; for there was great concern because of his degree of pigmentation and ''anyone with Hemochromatosis of such long standing has more than a fair chance of cirrhosis.'' It was a great relief when a liver biopsy revealed massive iron storage but no cirrhosis.

Throughout the treatment he remained chronically sore and stiff and says that, not matter how tired he is, only regular swimming can keep him mobile. He still has brown spots on his arms and the backs of his hands, and generally appears deeply tanned—despite the fact that he is seldom in the sun now—and continues to battle with general tiredness, never feeling completely well. When his hands finally became completely crippled, he underwent surgery for replacement of the affected knuckles.

HLA typing showed a daughter at risk. At 18 years of age, she had a transferrin saturation of 61%, 55% being the upper limit of normal. What will it show when she's 30?

* * *

To someone like me, who once believed that Hemochromatosis was only another word for Bronze Diabetes, the high incidence of joint disease has been a revelation. It crops up in almost every questionnaire and descriptions of the degree of resultant pain are to be found in nearly every letter; I can see the aching when these people walk towards me.

Arthritis in his fingers and impotence are what J.C. of Vancouver considers to have been his earliest indications. He now has diabetes, an enlarged liver, noticeable discolouration on feet and legs and "spider" veins on his face and upper chest. It was when his gall bladder was being removed that the "symptoms added up."

M.M. of Manitoba is one of the very few Hemochromatotics I have met who assures me that he has no vestige of bronzing. He had suffered, since the age of 29, with such severe, chronic indigestion, "heartburn and acid in the throat", that he could only sleep propped up on extra pillows. Then came soreness in hips, knees and lower legs, making walking a trial—which is a serious handicap for a farmer! Eight years later, during treatment for cancer on his nose, his blood was tested and high liver enzymes led to further tests for HH.

He is one of those who experienced "increased well-being" from the very first phlebotomy. His digestion has improved considerably. . . . but not the joint disease in hips and knees, or the soreness in the lower part of his legs; the high-pitched ringing in his ears is an irritation and torment of which others also complain. Merv's letters humorously report an improvement in his golf handicap. Since having two hip replacements he has been "wiping the floor with his opponents." Together with his wife, he recently organized the Hemochromatosis Awareness Week program in his area.

High liver enzymes led to May M's. diagnosis. She underwent the compulsory annual medical examination required in the government department in which she is employed, and finally found a reason for her joint stiffness, impaired memory and tiredness. Today she is overjoyed that a course of phlebotomies has restored her memory to normal and alleviated some of their other symptoms.

As a microbiologist, her job involves testing the blood of others, and I was surprised to learn from her that, as a Hemochromatotic, there are certain samples—for instance, those of persons thought to have Legionnaires disease—which she is not permitted to handle as her risk of contracting an infectious disease is higher than normal. What is particularly striking is that, since Dr. Margaret Krikker, President of the Hemochromatosis Research Foundation in the U.S.A., is especially interested to know what percentage of sufferers remembered being prone to recurrent infections, a question relating to this was included in the CHS questionnaire, at her request. Not one person replied in the affirmative. Is it possible then that people only *later* become subject to frequent colds and have little resistance to other infections? Would this occur only *after* the onset of the disease?

* * *

The list goes on and on. Pages could be written about people like J.G. of Cranbrook, B.C., who was afflicted with nausea and dizziness.—He says there is some improvement after five years of phlebotomy therapy but he still has to contend with high blood pressure, a bad liver, diabetes and arthritis.

And about Roy, who firmly believes that his iron overload (which was confirmed by a liver biopsy) was induced by a drug prescribed for gout, (although, in the beginning, he acknowledged that it could be a "what came first. . . the chicken or the egg?" kind of situation.)—Psuedo gout is one of the early symptoms experienced by countless others.

In due course, the blood iron level was reduced by phlebotomy therapy to the lower limit of the normal range, where it remains after four years.

When a Victoria physician could find no evidence of the original gout, treatment with the drug which, according to "The Essential Guide to Prescription Drugs:—James W. Long, M.D."—published by Harper and Row—may cause excessive accumulation of iron in body tissues if taken concurrently with iron preparations, was discontinued. Roy, however, remains sadly incapacitated and has been reduced, by arthritis, to using crutches. His story has taken an interesting twist. Roy was recently found to be a heterozygote—a carrier of one gene only!

He experiences bouts of atrial fibrillation and, although the condition has been bad enough to require hospitalization on several occasions—on one occasion electroconversion under anaesthetic—none of the doctors involved has been able to find a cause. He has been told that the condition is probably benign. Quite understandably, he remains curious about the effects of iron overload. His whole history poses a provocative question. Could the drug have increased a tendency to absorb iron from sources other than specific "iron preparations" because, being a carrier of HH he *has a pre-disposition to iron absorption*? Even if he only carries one gene?... And if so, what about carriers who are taking iron supplements?

Forms cannot paint pictures!

Questionnaires are all very well as far as statistics go. They provide data from which we learn, for example, that a very larger percentage of people who return them to us are of Scottish, English, Irish, French or Scandinavian descent. Just lately, we seem to have tracked down a growing number of Ukranian origin. The fact that the section headed "Physical findings at diagnosis" is seldom completed, might indicate that doctors have chosen not to pass on their findings to them. We may notice how frequently impotence and loss of libido crop up and that over 95% experienced some degree of weakness and fatigue in the early stages.—But forms are so CLINICAL! They state facts but do not communicate the despair and hopelessness felt by the people recording those facts! Very, very often an additional page is attached, or the back of the form will tell the true story... years and years of needless ill health; careers ruined; marriages destroyed. The desperation when it seems that no solution can be found.

What I have tried to set down, has not been extracted from questionnaires returned to the CHS. I have accumulated my information through direct contact or correspondence; these people have told their stories to **me**, personally, and I have included only what I have been given permission to repeat. I have heard the most incredible things... about excruciating abdominal pain and bleeding ulcers... about families with a history of rectal abscesses... about perspiration which smells "metallic" and breath that smells like "rust". I have checked this out (suspecting that this could be the characteristic "rotten apple" or "nailpolish" odour of the two extremes in badly managed diabetes) and it **does** smell like rust! They tell of blisters under rings when they are worn constantly, and of shirt cuffs turning green from some sort of reaction between sweat and metal watch straps; of rust-coloured semen and about the gilt trimmings which went green on the bed!... No form allows for disclosures concerning changes of personality... depression... anxiety.

Some degree of hearing loss is common enough to warrant special investigation.

Women

I have not been told by the husband of any severely Hemochromatotic wife whether or not they experience sexual problems, but a 55 year old woman who was diagnosed when she became concerned about the loss of body hair, admits to a markedly waning interest in sex. Because of her fortunate nature and bubbling personality, hers continues to be a happy marriage despite this. On the other hand, I know, from what women write to me, that wives of badly affected Hemochromatotic men can excuse impotence far more readily than lack of desire. They cannot endure "not being wanted!"

It is difficult to understand why there has to be so much unhappiness when a frank discussion would do much to alleviate the pain and stress for both spouses. "I can really relate to so much of what you said on CKNW," wrote a young wife during the 1987 Awareness Week. My husband has had nearly every symptom for nearly two years. In fact, we are now separated, due almost entirely to his condition. .... After months of pressuring him to, in turn, pressure his doctor to keep looking for a cause, I had reached the point where I couldn't handle it any longer. ... Now there is hope, perhaps!"

Sometimes true insight comes with the awful prospect of a beloved child suffering similarly in years to come; this puts things into a different perspective and makes the women more compassionate. But they do not say that this is easy!

There are those, whom I mentioned earlier, who are driven even to the lengths of dyeing their hair, believing that this would kindle a spark of interest, but I also know women who suffer from HH themselves, whose hair colour reflects some change in their systems; even to the extent that artificially lightened hair will not longer bleach to an ash blonde. It is strange, too, that—although in severe cases hair becomes wispy and of no particular colour—it seldom seems to go grey until iron stores are depleted.

While a proportion of women who have the genes do not have the disease, it should never be supposed that, when they do, they cannot be as severely afflicted by Hemochromatosis as their male counterparts are. Mrs. C's story is an excellent example, for she has had so many years of ill-health and still suffers cruelly.

After a complete hysterectomy in Montreal in 1974, she just could not regain normal strength; she became more and more exhausted and, a year later, bouts of diarrhea with cramps—which she had experienced in past years—returned; became worse and more frequent.

She was then living in Ontario, where a succession of doctors pronounced opinions varying from "just nerves... just depression" to "colitis and an irritable colon."

By the fall of 1981, she was hardly able to get up and dress herself. It became too difficult to concentrate and she had "pains everywhere, bloating, cramps and so on..!" The only nourishment she derived was from baby foods.

Finally, an endocrinologist in Toronto referred her to a gastroenterologist who, she says, "got down to business fast... had liver and bone marrow biopsies and iron studies done" which gave conclusive proof of Hemochromatosis.

Three years of phlebotomy therapy have undoubtedly saved her life but she does not enjoy the quality of life which should have been her due. The summer heat is unendurable, she is still very tired, has "many aches in the joints", has a "bloated feeling in the head" heavy, sore eyes (borderline glaucoma, too) and is generally unable to do very much. She does not know what it is to sleep really well and has had a rash on her face for two years—a complaint she shares with a good many of my other correspondents.

Alcohol

Since alcohol induced cirrhosis is one of the known causes of iron overload in secondary or non-inherited Hemochromatosis, victims of HH are continually having to defend themselves from too ready conclusions that this is the responsible factor in their illness. A young woman in her early twenties deplores this. "One can be as pure as the driven snow but no amount of protesting will convince some doctors that I'm not a secret drinker—of long standing!" A Calgary woman writes: "My father died of this iron disease and they say it's because he drank too much beer!"... Which could have been the case, but I sincerely hope her physician does not leave it at that!

Another cry of protest; this time from Northern British Columbia. "The specialist first believed that my brother's liver problem was caused by alcohol and ignored his insistence that he didn't drink enough for this to be the case! Unfortunately, here in the North, there is a high alcohol consumption and you can be put into a general category unless they come to realize that the diagnosis is incorrect!"

Much has been written on the subject of alcohol and iron absorption and in cases of established homozygosity or diagnosed HH, patients are generally warned, because of possible liver damage, against heavy alcohol consumption. They are told especially to avoid red wine. There is, however, only one case in my own records, of regular usage before the onset of the disease. Some mention a history of alcoholism in previous generations.

Oh, that terrible tiredness!

If one of the more frequent first indications was "not feeling right", the most constant cry, before **and** after treatment must certainly be "I'm so tired!" Asked what symptoms remain unchanged, a man from Wheatley, Ontario wrote cryptically: "Tired!.... Tired!.... Tired!"

This fatigue has to be seen to be believed. Very few are spared this. To a Hemochromatotic person, carrying on with a job usually means going to work and coming home; collapsing into the nearest chair—perhaps to doze. Early to bed, to sleep, in order to be able to get up and make it back to work again next day. The most ordinary undertakings, like shopping, can be an ordeal. It is not unusual to give up at the supermarket if the standing becomes too much; a list to jog the memory is essential—if one remembers to take that list!

Something almost superhuman keeps them going. I would dearly like to know the origin of the metaphor "a man of iron"; for certainly, many have needed to be very strong in order to have survived the onslaughts of the disease. Nine years after having to retire, my husband has returned to full-time work and will not stop although he comes home grey with pain and with hands too swollen to take his keys out of his pocket. Every ounce of energy is conserved so that his performance at his job might surpass that of normal men, half his age.

"Women of iron" exist too. How some of them cope with housework, young children and the enervating process of phlebotomies is astounding. But male or female, the indomitable will must inevitably be undermined by periods of chronic, insurmountable weakness and fatigue. It is particularly hard on young people like G.H.

I first heard about him from his aunt, who wrote to me after I had appeared on television with my husband as my "Exhibit A" and, for once, since the producers of the show had not seen fit to cap my performance with a comment by some expert, I was not shot down in flames with the usual statements about "one in twenty thousand!" At that stage I still hoped that my daughter's case might be unique and that other young people would not be similarly affected. Deeply moved though I was by what G.'s aunt told me about him, I could not believe that such colossal iron overload could have been encountered in one so young, in his early thirties, and with a wife and three young sons to support.

Before his diagnosis, he had been visibly unwell for approximately three years. His symptoms were mainly pain and stiffness in arms, legs, hands and feet and, although he had gradually been losing body hair, he was not aware of this until the hair began to grow back after treatment. There were several visits to his doctor during his period and X-rays were taken but no reason could be found for his discomfort; towards the end of the three years, his movements resembled those of a very old man.

When it was found that his liver was slightly enlarged, he was referred to a specialist in internal medicine, who, after about four months of investigation, scheduled a liver biopsy.

The week before he was due to go into hospital, G. began to manifest symptoms of diabetes which, unfortunately he did not mention to the physician—although he did tell the nurse who came to do the routine checks which preceded the biopsy—but it is still remarkable that his, by then very evident diabetes, was not detected.

After he was discharged from the hospital, both he and his wife "naively assumed that he was so very sick as a result of the biopsy and that it would soon subside." When his vision began to blur and he became increasingly disoriented, however, his wife took him back to the doctor. Diabetes was confirmed and when the results of the biopsy became available, both the family doctor and the specialist sought to find a reason for the high iron content in his liver. "Within a few days they came to believe that it was this rare condition known as Hemochromatosis." Today those doctors are more than aware that the disorder is not rare, and are extremely well informed on the subject of iron overload.

Life has not been easy for G. The iron has affected his liver, pancreas, endocrine glands and various bones and joints. Some of the damage is irreversible, but he has coped with a long course of bleeds—initially two a week—and continues to work at a job which involves some very heavy work. Considering the fatigue he has to fight, every inch of the way, what he accomplishes is extraordinary. Because of HLA and other tests, he knows that one of his sisters has HH and another is a carrier. His children will be very carefully watched.

CHAPTER FIVE

The vital importance of early detection.

THERE IS THE MOST INCREDIBLE SATISFACTION IN LEARN-
ing of the increasing awareness across Canada. One hears of
knowledgeable doctors in Quebec and Ontario, at hospitals like
the Women's College Hospital in Toronto and the Victoria Hospital in London; in Edmonton, Calgary and Winnipeg; New
Westminster, and smaller centres in every province. The disease
has a high profile in British Columbia, at the Vancouver General
and Saint Paul's Hospitals, and at UBC, in many departments;
for instance, since joint disease is such a common complication
in HH, iron overload is suspected and relevant blood tests carried
out whenever anyone under 50 presents with chondrocalcinosis—
calcium deposits in the cartilege. In Newfoundland a large scale
program which involves the screening of people in high-risk
groups is under way at the moment.

A man on Vancouver Island, will outdance anyone at a party,
in spite of almost crippling arthritis and weekly phlebotomies.
But then, he has been spared other complications, like the inevitable fatigue and weakness, by prompt diagnosis of his underlying complaint. The possibility that his pain and stiffness
might be due to Hemochromatosis was recognised by a doctor at
the arthritis clinic in Vancouver and confirmed at the University
of British Columbia Health Sciences Hospital. It is regrettable
that he seems to encounter such difficulty in arranging for
venesection back in his home town.

Mrs. D.W. is an Island resident who passes on only good

news. She has arthritis and hypertension but was unaware of any other symptoms which could have indicated a more serious problem. She writes, "Thank God I had—and still have — a sagacious doctor in Dr. M.B who, after having blood work done on me, sent me to Dr. R.W. with his findings! A few of the usual tests were done and topped off with a biopsy."

As gratifying as these examples of detection may be, however, the effects are lasting. When the victim is not known to be related to a known proband, to achieve early diagnosis is difficult. Even the very first indications appear too late. There are no symptoms or signs of body iron overload until iron loading is well established and, even in the late stages of the disease, it may be overlooked because it presents in the form of diabetes, arthritis, impotence, liver or cardiac disease.

While an increasing number of potential victims are being pinpointed by family screening and the diagnostic record improves, the flip side of the coin still comes up too often. There are countless cases of "face-value" misdiagnosis—liver involvement as chronic hepatitis, for instance —or the presenting manifestation is accepted without anyone asking "why?"... How many people resign themselves to the fact that they have sudden onset diabetes without ever probing deeper. **We** asked: "Why, why, why?"—For six years no-one could tell us, but **now** we know!

Stories like the one related by E.S. of Wenatchee, Washington are heart-warming but far too rare. Nevertheless, if the best news is that concerning discovery **before** damage has been done, it is still wonderful to be told about someone who was spotted before there were any warning signs and therefore earlier than is the general rule. E.S. had that experience and has a a most incredible story to relate. His iron overload was found quite by chance.

A scientist, he works at a research centre with both a government department and Washington State University. One of the men from WSU had taken advantage of a health evaluation program offered by the Seventh Day Adventist church, and was so impressed with the testing that he asked if this could be done at the centre, if enough people were interested.

"Fortunately," says E.S., "we had more than enough for them to make a visit. Since these people do not eat meat, they routinely screen for iron in their blood tests. The screening done here at the regular clinic does not include iron unless requested by a doctor.'' As is the case in Canada, ''the philosphy is, or at least was, that there is nothing to be gained and most people would not benefit from the cost.''

When the results were returned and discussed, E.S. noticed that his iron was ''off scale on the high side (serum iron about 260). I took this information with me to the clinic when I went for my physical and the blood series was repeated and found to be correct. Fortunately, again, the MD's here are in close contact with the University of Washington and Doctor Finch—who was at UW then —is, as you are aware, a leading authority on Hemochromatosis.''

What interested the physicians concerned, was that E.S. was 55 years old with no symptoms other than high serum iron and a ruddy complexion. A liver biopsy ''clinched'' HH. Hemosiderin was apparent in many cells, there was some scarring and the liver may have been slightly enlarged although the liver function tests were normal.

He is a lucky man and he knows it. He was so thankful for having found out about his iron overload before symptoms appeared, that he ''volunteered himself as a research subject for Dr. Clem Finch.''

It might be Hemochromatosis!

That the medical profession frequently overlook important clues is not necessarily due to incompetence. The disease has simply been accorded too low a profile and, too often, the patient can only say, ''I just don't feel right!''

It is understandable that the physician should look for clinical evidence before forming an opinion—a million appendices would have been removed on countless occasions if doctors had been swayed by the patients' own diagnosis of what ailed them —but until every potential Hemochromatotic can be found by some, feasible, routine program (perhaps such as that envisaged by the Hemochromatosis Research Foundation, in which blood donors would be screened with the co-operation of the Red Cross) the only solution seems to lie in an awareness campaign; until seemingly insignificant symptoms are programmed somehow into the diagnostic procedure of every family doctor.

For some years I was consumed with bitterness as I considered the havoc wreaked by Hemochromatosis in my own family. Every time I re-lived the years of needless suffering which my husband had to endure before the correct diagnosis saved his life; when I thought of a wonderful career cut short at its peak; when I saw hands that once held crowds enthralled, no longer able to play beautiful music without the accompaniment of groans of pain; when I became conscious of the tilt of the head which comes when not only the gift of perfect pitch has been taken away but it has obviously become a strain to follow a conversation—let alone catch the punch lines in a good television show —I railed at the callousness and negligence which we appeared to have suffered at the hands of the medical profession. My opinion of doctors as a breed ranged from hero-worship of the researchers and those who had discovered the underlying cause of what ailed Tom, to admiration for any physician who knew about Hemochromatosis, and contempt for one who did not.

As a result of my study, I still have little patience with doctors who do not read what has been written by the experts, and stories like the one about the "bronzed" woman on Vancouver Island, who was given iron shots to "pick her up" when she was so weak from iron overload that she could no longer climb the stairs, raise my blood pressure. However, I have heard enough now to know that it is possible for the most perceptive physician to overlook the wood for the trees.

Mrs.D., a doctor's wife, the mother of a registered nurse and with her own, long career in nursing now behind her, remembers that, while outsiders were concerned, neither she nor anyone else in her family noticed vital signs. "On looking back, I was weak and unsteady for four years. Friends questioned my poor colour but I was not aware of it." When she had a bad fall, she was jaundiced "to a bronze tan" and, while she did not feel too ill, she realized that something must have caused her to fall; that there had to be a reason for her dizziness, unsteady gait and confusion. This became more obvious when she had a second fall. A temporary diagnosis was made but rejected when she showed no improvement.

She was in a coma for four days after being re- admitted to hospital, with abdominal distention and swelling of the limbs. Sadly, she showed little improvement after some years of treatment and felt that her condition was too "far advanced". Besides having to use a cane, she complained, until her death, of general weakness— her voice remained weak, shaky hands made writing difficult and she reported that she had been left with a poor memory.

It has overwhelmed and humbled me to discover how many medical practitioners have shared our experience. I literally wept over the letter from Dr. L., in which he described how he, himself, had been forced to retire from practice because of severe joint disease caused by Hemochromatosis. A surgeon at a leading Canadian university, he had seen only two proven cases, both of which came to autopsy. In December of 1968 he suffered his first coronary occlusion. In January 1974, after returning from the annual meeting of a prominent medical association, he started to vomit and did so for the next 36 hours. He was admitted, semi-comatosed, to hospital where tests showed his liver enzymes raised, as a result of which a liver biopsy was performed.

"For eighteen months prior to that date," he told me, "I had been having regular tests done because I didn't feel right. These tests showed a gradual but steady deterioration of kidney and liver function and I knew my joints were so bad that I would have to quit in the middle of an operation and soak my hands in hot water."

On repeated examination by his colleagues he was told, "We cannot account for these findings." He has never worked again. What happened after that, he tells in this way: " When Dr. B. came in the following evening to tell me the results of the biopsy, he said, 'Dr. L., have you heard of Hemochromatosis?'

" I raised myself up and said: 'Good God, Boy, that's an autopsy finding!' He then stated, 'Not this time, Sir!' "

The doctor started on phlebotomies and then developed angina, which resulted in his being re-admitted to the Coronary Care Unit. "It became a vicious circle.... on recovery, more phlebotomies.... then more chest pain... and so on."

By the fall of 1974, he says, life had become a "full time maintenance job!" However, by December of that year, 25,540 cc's of blood had been removed during about 50 bleeds; the amount and the frequency depended on whether or not he was in heart failure at the time.

Two or three years ago, he thought he was beginning to feel somewhat better. The decision that he would never practise again had been made long before that. Then he had another coronary but thinks that, having recovered from that and bouts of vomiting for several months, he is "quite a bit better" but the joints are "terrible!" In reply to my emotional outburst of "Why should this have happened to someone like **you?**" the simple reply was: "Why not?"

* * *

On the diagnosis of Hemochromatosis, Dr. L. has this to say:
"The doctor thinks, 'The patient has something wrong;
I don't know what is wrong;
It might be Hemochromatosis...
I will order the necessary tests!'"

REFERENCES

(1)   Saddi R, Feingold J: Idiopathic Hemochromatosis: an autosomal recessive disease. Clin. Genet. 5: 234-241, 1974
        Simon M, Bourel M, et al: Idiopathic Hemochromatosis. Demonstration of recessive transmission and early detection by family HLA typing. N Eng J Med 297: 1017-1021, 1977

(ii)   Dadone M M et al: Hereditary Hemochromatosis: Am J Clin Path 78: 196-207, 1982

(iii)   S T Borwein, C N Ghent, P R FLanagan, M J Chamberlain and L S Valberg: Genetic and Phenotypic Expression of Hemochromatosis in Canadians: Clinical and Investigative Medicine (Vol 6, no 3, pp 171-179, 1983

(iv)   Sheldon J H: Haemochromatosis: New York, Oxford University Press, 1935

(v)   Mark L Bassett, MB Ch B; June W Halliday, Ph D; Lawrie W Powell, MD PhD Hemochromatosis—Newer Concepts: Diagnosis and Management; Year Book Medical Publishers Inc, 1980

(vi)   Corwin Q. Edwards et al: Hereditary Hemochromatosis—Diagnosis in Siblings and Children: New Eng J of Med: 7-12, July 1977

(vii)   Motulsky A G: Genetics of Hemochromatosis: N Eng J Med 301:1291, 1979

Cox T M: Prevalence of the hemochromatosis gene: N Eng J Med 302: 695-696, 1980

(viii) Bothwell T H; Charlton R W; Motulsky A G: Idiopathic Hemochromatosis: Stanbury J et al: The Metabolic Basis of Inherited Disease: Mc Graw Hill, 1983.

(ix) Blood, Pure and Eloquent. Maxwell M. Wintrobe M.D., Ph.D.,M.A.C.P. Hon. D.Sc. Mc Graw-Hill Book Company, 1980.

(x) Milder S M; Cook J D; Stray S; and Finch C A: Idiopathic Hemochromatosis, an Interim Report: Medicine vol 59 no 1, 1980

(xi) Disler P B; Lynch S R; Charlton R W; Torrance J D; Bothwell T H; Walker R B; and Mayet F: The effect of tea on iron absorption: Gut. 1975, 16, 193-200

(xii) Callender S T; Marney S R; Warner G T: Eggs and iron absorption: Brit J of Haem, 19: 657-665, 1970

(xiii) Rajantie et al—1893. Scandinavian Journal of Haematol. 31: 20-22

(xiv) "The HLA linked iron loading gene in an Afrikaner population." Meyer, Ballot, Bothwell et al. Brit. Journal of Med. Gen. 1987, 24: 348-356

For further information please write to:
The Canadian Hemochromatosis Society
Box 94303
Richmond, B.C.
V6Y 2A6

The writer is indebted to Dr. Margaret Krikker, President of the Hemochromatosis Research Foundation, and to Roberta Crawford, President of the Iron Overload Diseases Association, Inc., for permission to quote from "Hemochromatosis Awareness" and "Ironic Blood" respectively.